ABOUT THE A

Victor Zorza was born in Poland in 1925 and came to England via Russia during World War Two. After service with the RAF he joined the BBC, and then became the *Guardian*'s correspondent on Communist affairs and on East-West relations, writing a syndicated column which appeared in leading newspapers around the world. He received the Journalist of the Year Award for 'predicting with astonishing accuracy and against the flow of informed opinion' the invasion of Czechoslovakia in 1968.

Rosemary Zorza was born in England in 1923, served in the Army during the war, and worked for the BBC afterwards. Later she became a potter. She has published a book, *Pottery for Pleasure*, and also teaches. The Zorzas now divide their time between England and the USA, where Victor Zorza writes a column for the *Washington Post*. Their brief account of what the hospice had done for their daughter appeared in the *Washington Post* and in The *Guardian*, stimulating great interest in the hospice movement on both sides of the Atlantic. Victor and Rosemary Zorza are now co-chairmen of the National Advisory Council of the National Hospice Organisation in the USA. (An afterword gives a note on the hospice movement and a list of hospices in Great Britain.)

A Way to Die
Living to the end
ROSEMARY and VICTOR ZORZA

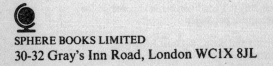

SPHERE BOOKS LIMITED
30-32 Gray's Inn Road, London WC1X 8JL

First published in Great Britain by André Deutsch Ltd 1980
Copyright © Victor Zorza and Rosemary Zorza 1980
Published by Sphere Books Ltd 1981

Printed and bound in Great Britain by
©ollins, Glasgow

To W. J. Weatherby

Without whose friendship, encouragement and help this book would not have been written

AUTHORS' NOTE: Our thanks are due to the hospice staff not only for their help during Jane's illness, but also for sharing with us so frankly their recollections of those days. Some of the people who appear in these pages have asked that they should not be identified, and we have therefore, for the sake of consistency, changed all names except those of members of Jane's family.

Prologue

'I don't want to die,' our daughter Jane said, when she learned at the age of twenty-five that she had cancer. But in the months which followed she proved that dying need not be the dread experience most of us imagine. Far from being the defeat it is usually thought to be, her death was a kind of victory – a battle won against pain and terror. It was a shared triumph for Jane and for those who worked to help her, and especially for a new British approach to the care of the dying.

We hesitated when it was first suggested that she should go to a hospice. We dared not risk experimenting, at her life's end, with new approaches to dying. But we soon found that there was nothing experimental about the hospice which took her in. It was part of the National Health Service, whose facilities are available free of charge to all patients. The hospice was located in the grounds of one of Oxford University's teaching hospitals. Jane would be in good hands.

Afraid of pain like all of us, Jane had a horror of the nothingness that she believed death to be, a conviction that neither science nor religion could do anything for her. But Jane's arrival at the hospice was a turning point; it enabled her to carry out the most difficult act of her life with ease and tranquillity. What might have been an appalling and shattering experience was made as easy as possible both for her and for us. She met her end surrounded by love, with all emotional debts paid and the pattern of her life complete. For us the memory is not one of pain and anguish but of her calm smile and peace of mind. She was ready for what she knew must come, accepting it with a serenity that belied her early fears.

This is what the hospice did for Jane, and for us – for it treats the family as a unit – and what it can do for all the people who turn to it for help. She urged us to write about the hospice so that others might benefit from our experience. 'There should be more hospices, everyone should know about them,' she said. She hoped that the pain and fear so many of us dread might be alleviated as hers had been.

When we told Jane's story to our friends, they responded by relating to us their own experiences with dying relatives and friends, and often these would be accounts of terrible physical and mental distress – of loneliness, fear and rejection in hospitals that had no facilities or time for the dying. They spoke of the sadness and guilt that build up when words are left unsaid until it is too late. 'It was different for you,' they said. 'Jane must have been an extraordinary person.' We were uneasily aware of the impression of heroic saintliness our account of Jane's last days might convey. Jane was no paragon, and our friends knew it. But should we write about this for strangers? Should we tell them of the family stress and friction which preceded our discovery of the hospice? We reminded ourselves that every family is subject to its own tensions when someone dies, and that it might help others to know how ours were resolved.

Then someone said, 'You should write about it just as you've told me.' And that's what we did.

The article we wrote appeared in the *Guardian* and the Washington *Post*, and then in many other newspapers round the world. We were overwhelmed by the response: more than ten thousand letters from readers who wanted further information on what hospices do, where they can be found, how they could be established; about Jane, and what made it possible for her to cope as she did; and about our own experience as a family. We went back to England to work on the book. We had lived in Washington for nearly ten years, spending only the summers in England, where Jane had remained to attend university and then to become a teacher. Her older brother Richard had gone to America on a scholarship and had stayed on. We made our home in

Washington because Victor, who was writing a syndicated column for the Washington *Post*, needed to be there. Now he put the column aside, and Rosemary gave up the pottery that had been her main occupation since the children grew up. We talked to the hospice doctors and staff, who gave us their recollections of Jane's stay there and of their conversations with her. We spoke to Jane's friends. We relived the last five months of Jane's illness. It wasn't easy. But whenever we struck a bad patch, we would say to each other: Remember the hospice. And then we were ready to write.

Chapter 1

It began one July morning in 1975.

We were spending the summer at our English home, Dairy Cottage, in a Buckinghamshire village. At twenty-three, our very independent daughter Jane had settled nearby, in an old cottage where farm workers had once lived.

That morning Rosemary walked through the beautiful English countryside to call on Jane. It was a peaceful scene, and she stopped to enjoy the sights and sounds of the fields.

When she came into the cottage, she found Jane already up, padding about the old, uneven floors in bare feet; she never wore shoes at home. Then Jane held up her right foot to be inspected. 'What do you think of that, Mum?'

Her tone was so casual that Rosemary looked down with a smile, assuming Jane was in one of her joking moods. Her smile faded at what she saw. There was an ugly, puffy, black-purple lump about the size of a small coin just above her middle toe.

'Looks a bit strange,' Rosemary said. 'Have you had it long?'

Jane hesitated, then replied slowly, 'I'm not sure. It was just a mole before it began to grow.'

Rosemary, always sensitive to her daughter's feelings, was aware then of the deep concern under Jane's calm front. 'I think you should see Dr. Sullivan,' she said gently.

She expected an argument, but Jane blurted out, 'He says I'll have to go to hospital to have it taken off.'

Rosemary studied the expressive, attractive face, sometimes that of a sophisticated woman, sometimes still that of a young girl. It wasn't like Jane to consult the family doctor without saying anything. She looked again at the black-purple spot. It couldn't be anything to worry about, surely, such a small spot, a long way from the vital parts of the body – heart, lungs, eyes . . .

'I had a blemish like that near my ear, remember?' she said. 'They just nicked it off in a minute or two.'

'Would you mind coming with me when I go?' Jane asked. 'Hospitals are such a bore.'

That, too, wasn't like Jane. Since she had grown up, she always asserted her independence. Rosemary began to worry.

At the hospital, Jane went in alone to see the doctor. She had been irritated at having to wait nearly an hour before her turn came. She was bitterly critical of a badly organised system that wasted so much of people's time. She went in at last very angry. She came out in tears.

'He says I must have two days in hospital.'

The little seed of fear began to grow. 'Did he say anything else?'

'They'll take tests.' She looked at Rosemary with frightened eyes. 'When I asked him if he thought it was cancer, he said that was a word he didn't use.'

Cancer. They had both considered the same possibility.

Jane didn't say anything more, but that night she wrote in her diary: 'The fact that I've got a "growth" that could presumably be cancerous terrifies me. For a short time I had a really horrible thought of me dying and how I would come to terms with the prospect of it happening soon. It's very unlikely to be anything even vaguely serious.'

When she was admitted to the local hospital a week later, Jane was appalled to find she would have to stay there for a week after the operation. They would cut out the black spot, they told her, and take an area of skin from her thigh to graft over the wound. It would be ten days before the test results were known.

Skin grafts are painful, Jane discovered, and operations on the foot especially painful. She hadn't been warned, she complained; but in spite of the pain, she refused to take the Valium that was part of her medication. She didn't want to be tranquillised. She wrote in her diary: 'It's amazing (not really!) how, when one is treated like a child, one begins to feel and react like one. I want to revolt against the pettiness of this existence and the way one is treated as an object.'

She had been told she would have to stay in for a week after the operation. The next day she reported angrily to us: 'Now they say ten days. Why can't they make up their minds?' Always the news was bad. Finally the doctor told her that another operation might be necessary if the test results were 'nasty'. Jane's friends worked hard with us to help her pass the boring and anxious hours, but her spirits were often low. She feared the news would be bad – and so did we.

On the tenth day we were in the garden trying to enjoy the sunshine when the phone rang. It wasn't Jane, but the woman in the next bed. 'Jane's too upset to talk,' she said. There was a pause, then she added: 'The doctor's just told her that the growth was malignant. It's cancer.'

We hurried over to the hospital. By then, Jane was calmer. She'd been half expecting it, she told us. 'I can come out tomorrow to fatten up for the next op.' The news was not all grim, there was reason for hope. It was skin cancer, and might not recur. Her chances were no worse than those of anybody else – no worse than the likelihood of her getting it in the first place.

'Of course,' the ward sister told us, 'no doctor can sign a blank cheque for health . . .'

'Of course not,' we agreed.

The next consultation with the specialists yielded better news. Another operation wouldn't be necessary after all – a sufficiently large area of tissue had already been removed. There was no need to go further.

The anxiety began to subside and everyone felt a sense of anti-climax. We'd made a terrible fuss about nothing very much. All that was necessary was to help Jane build up her strength.

She came home to recover. Now, knowing that it would pass, she could cope with the pain. If she had any further worries about the cancer reappearing, she kept them to herself.

Richard, who was in Boston, urged us to find out everything we could about what kind of cancer it was. His American fiancée, Joan, had a relative who'd suffered from a severe form of skin cancer. Perhaps this was similar; we should get as many details as possible. But we brushed him aside. What the doctors had said sounded good to us. Why worry unnecessarily?

We had always tended to worry too much over Jane. From her childhood on she'd been vulnerable, in spite of her determination to 'go it alone' – or perhaps because of it. Signs of her strength of mind were apparent early in life. The baby who cried so loudly, and so often, grew into the child who questioned authority, who insisted on doing things her own way, preferring to make her own mistakes.

As a girl growing up in England, she had retreated into writing poetry whose tragic intensity contrasted strangely with her mild, neat appearance. But her will power wasn't equalled by a strong constitution, and she would often expect her body to do more than it could. She needed to be protected from herself.

Jane might have got what she wanted by smiling and being charming; she had the looks for it. More importantly, she had whatever it is that attracts others, the quality that turns heads in the street. When she was an infant, strangers wanted to hold the pretty baby; later they would try to get the toddler to smile that sudden, beaming smile. But Jane became sparing with her smiles: she would inherit her generation's fear of 'phoniness' to an intense degree.

As she grew older, the pattern was the same. She began to look below the surface and reject what came too easily. School days are hard for the non-conformist, the questioner. Idealists are inevitably frustrated as they pursue their dreams, perfectionists always disappoint themselves by not meeting their own standards. Jane never believed in her own successes; she only recognised the failures. She tried to express her realities in her poems, but rarely showed them to anyone. Like all children, she played and fought and made jokes when life was good, but she also suffered deep fits of depression during which nobody could reach her. As she grew older, she tried harder to overcome these brooding moods, but never quite succeeded. These were times of despair about the world, coupled with great self-doubt, times when any criticism of her seemed overwhelming and any encouragement was resented as an attempt at consolation. As with all of us, Jane's reactions varied as the different sides of her character were called upon to face particular situations. She wasn't one to give up or to circumvent. The easy road, the majority view, were not for her; and yet the impression this conveys of a stern, unwavering realist is too strong. Her decisions weren't always so sharply defined, so absolute. She dithered, she agonized, often she changed her mind. Always there were questions, and then she would question the answers she was given. Not afraid of being different, she never thought of herself as a strong person in spite of her definite opinions.

In her teens these opinions became even firmer, and she learned to keep the self-doubts hidden. She dropped poetry for politics. She became a committed rebel, perpetually at war with her father, whose liberal views she found too mild. Victor hoped she would recognise that he was taking her seriously by arguing with her as adult to adult, but their discussions were often disastrous. She had no patience with his professionally polished, ordered and informed brand of argument, and usually stamped off in a rage rather than awaiting the conclusion of the argument.

Sometimes her sense of humour came to the rescue and she would manage to have the last word with a well-timed exit line. It was the period when student agitation over Vietnam and other issues was attracting world-wide attention. Jane came back from the most recent demonstration bursting with righteous indignation and a secret delight that she found hard to conceal. She had even been trampled by a police horse! Three young American girls were staying with the family, and Victor said angrily: 'Jane, on no account are you to take those girls to the next demo!' Jane answered sweetly: 'Dad, I shall only be showing our American guests the sights of London.'

When Jane graduated with a degree in social science, she

decided that teaching was the profession that would give her a chance to work at the three things she wanted to do most – contribute to the struggle for a better world, spend a lot of time with children, and travel. Although she never lost her awareness of social problems, she soon grew disillusioned with politics and concentrated on a more private life. She became a vegetarian long before it was popular or even accepted. She studied her diet scientifically, struggling to convert us to a more healthy way of eating. She gave up smoking, repeatedly. She began to garden seriously. Now she didn't listen only to the music of the counter-culture, of rebellion and freedom. She discovered that she could listen to the classics without feeling she was betraying her generation.

Jane wanted love, but when it came she found it hard to accept completely, difficult to give up her freedom absolutely – and so she would drive her lover away, only to wish him back when loneliness set in. Finally she decided that she had to prove to herself she could survive alone, that she couldn't call herself free while she depended on another's company.

Her relationship with Victor had never recovered completely from the difficult years of her adolescence. She tried to make things up with him, but there were many setbacks. It was too easy for them to misunderstand each other. The years of puppy fat and its attendant miseries were over for Jane; she had learned to keep her figure under control. Yet although beginning to realise she was attractive, she was still vulnerable beneath the surface poise. In spite of her firm opinions and a sturdy, nonconformist sense of independence, she could also collapse in confusion and uncertainty.

We knew that Jane's experience of cancer would increase this vulnerability. We were relieved to learn that the disease was not of the deadly variety, but then came a new cause for anxiety: Jane wasn't getting her strength back. The summer was over and we had to go back to America. Jane tried to return to her old routine, but the journey to the school and the job of teaching were tiring. She was ill with a number of minor ailments that winter. Often she couldn't carry out in class the work she'd prepared so thoroughly the day before.

It would be better to work at a school nearer home. She decided to give up her job and look for another.

But the timing was wrong. There were twenty thousand unemployed teachers in England that year. The spring passed, we came home for another summer, and still she'd found nothing. The constant rejections had affected her self-confidence; she grew seriously worried about her future. At last she was accepted for the job of teaching the children of three middle-class families in Greece – not the kind of work her social conscience demanded, but by now anything was welcome. And she liked Greece.

After months of worry and indecision, Jane found relief in action. She terminated the lease on her cottage. She harvested her vegetable crop and disposed of potatoes, onions, carrots, beets, and homemade wine. She sorted and re-sorted her possessions, regretting that she had so many belongings when life should be kept simple. She packed, stored and gave away. She complained of chaos, but worked in an orderly way, making neat lists of tasks to be done. It was sad to leave a place where she'd often been happy and had gained the confidence to live alone. But it was time for a new life.

She flew off to Athens on a dark, wet night in September after a celebration dinner with us. That evening we were happy and relaxed together. She and Victor were closer than they'd been for years.

Jane was good at keeping in touch by letter. We learned she was settling down in Greece, making friends, and longing for the summer when she would visit the islands and spend time in the mountains. She sounded happy – a new Jane – and we dared to hope she had completely recovered.

Then one February weekend we were on a hiking trip in the Virginia hills. Rosemary had gone to have coffee with friends when Victor suddenly burst in on them and began to talk compulsively, almost incoherently. They couldn't grasp what he was saying . . . something about Jane and cancer?

'I've booked you on the plane home tonight,' he said.

That got through. It was as if the word 'cancer' was a hammer blow that had smashed the pattern of our lives into little pieces. Victor hadn't spoken directly to Jane. Richard's fiancée, Joan, had taken Jane's phone call and passed a message on to Richard, who had tracked us down with some difficulty. But Jane hadn't yet been able to share her feelings with any of her immediate family. We tried desperately to phone her in Greece over and over again, but there was no reply.

We drove back to Washington through the waning light of a sunlit but bitterly cold day. The mountains in the distance were a deep blue, but we hardly noticed them. Our thoughts were far away.

Halfway to the city we tried to phone Jane again from a booth in a vacant car lot. While we waited, the wind whipped a plastic cup round and round in circles. Time seemed to stand still in that lonely spot. At last we heard Jane's voice, crackling over the long, long distance between Greece and America.

'I'm on my way to England. You don't have to come,' she said at first. But when she heard that Rosemary had already decided to meet her in England, the relief flooded her voice. 'Terrific!' She added more cheerfully, 'See you tomorrow, then.'

In Washington Rosemary tried to pack, to leave the house in order. But the familiar objects felt strange in this context of utter disorganisation and chaos. The pattern of life seemed lost.

The news was certainly bad. A week before, Jane had woken up to find a lump in her groin. Her first thought was that this was the place the doctors always looked when she went for a checkup. She remembered there had been days in the past few weeks when she'd felt really ill, and decided to see the local doctor. He told her there was nothing to worry about – something was wrong, but it wasn't a return of the cancer. A few days later she checked with another doctor. This time the response was very different. 'Go back to England immediately, to the hospital where they operated on you.'

Rosemary reached London first. Dairy Cottage had been

rented to tenants until the end of May, so she had arranged to stay with friends in town. But she rang the family doctor in the country and described what had happened.

'Bring Jane straight here from the airport,' he told her. 'If the plane's late, I'll wait in the surgery.' Julian Sullivan, a calm, unflappable man, was businesslike but sympathetic on the phone. And Jane liked him – that would be a help.

She arrived at London Airport dressed in blue jeans and a bright Indian waistcoat with a scarf knotted, pirate-fashion, round her head. She looked so happy to be home again that for a moment the nightmare was almost forgotten. But her confidence soon started slipping away.

When we reached the doctor's small waiting room in the village near Dairy Cottage, we were told to go straight in. 'Will you come with me, Mum?' Jane asked. 'I might need a bit of support.'

Yet she faced him cheerfully enough. Here was someone she had come to like and trust over the many years he had looked after the family. She knew, too, that he would be frank with her.

Dr. Sullivan, in a neat dark suit, shook hands, smiling at her, his eyes warm. 'Let's see what we can do for you, Jane,' he said.

The examination took only a moment. The small white lump in Jane's groin was plainly visible. Dr. Sullivan didn't try to hide his concern. It looked like a tumour in the lymphatic gland, and would have to come out, he told her.

'I've already booked you a bed in the local hospital,' he added. 'You must be there by nine o'clock tomorrow morning.'

'Could it be malignant?' Jane asked, her nervousness beginning to show, though she still half-hoped that she was wrong.

Yes, he said, it probably was, but of course he couldn't be sure.

If she had it cut out, would that cure it?

No, other tumours might grow and they would have to be removed, too.

Jane swore, then burst into tears. Rosemary and the doctor watched her helplessly. With shaking hands, she lit a cigarette and puffed furiously. Then she crushed it out in the spotless wash basin and, realising what she'd done, began to apologise.

'There's nothing to apologise for, Jane,' Dr. Sullivan said gently. 'I know how you feel. I had a lump removed a few years ago. It is a big shock.' He gave her time to pull herself together while he talked reassuringly. But as she walked back through the waiting room, the other patients looked sympathetically at her.

'Let's get out of here,' she said.

We drove back through the darkness and rush-hour traffic along the familiar road to London. There had been so many rides along this road in the past, to theatres, parties, boating trips; to school, exams. Never had any journey been under such a shadow as this one.

That night there was a reunion in the friends' house where we were staying, all of us laughing and talking over a good supper eaten with the wine that Jane had brought from Greece. She spoke a little of cancer, but managed to keep the nightmare well in the background until it was time for bed. There the fears were waiting for her. The pain of another operation, the threat of more lumps appearing . . .

Jane took some Valium and managed to sleep.

By nine-thirty the next morning we were at the hospital waiting for X-rays to be taken. She was in good spirits, and trying to count her blessings. She was glad to be home, she had contacted some friends and was looking forward to further reunions. She knew she would get the best treatment and that cancer patients had priority. All her treatments would be free under the National Health Service.

After Jane had been X-rayed, she walked to a little room to wait for the operation.

The surgeon was a small, fierce-looking man, with no warmth or comfort in his eyes, who did not seem capable of the God-like task of cutting into living flesh. When he came out of Jane's room after his pre-operative examination, urgent, tense, he glared at Rosemary. 'And who are you?'

She wanted to snap back but decided not to make cracks at the surgeon who was about to cut into her daughter. She said merely that she was Jane's mother.

His manner didn't change. He told her tersely he would operate that afternoon to remove the lymph gland. He seemed to regard the human body purely as a machine that had to be put right. Mechanics don't have to be polite to the machines they repair. What did it matter as long as he mended Jane's body?

Rosemary went home to wait, as is usual in England, although she preferred the American custom of remaining in the hospital while an operation is in progress. When she telephoned the hospital later that evening, she was told that the operation had been successful and Jane was comfortable. Such reports are always superficial. Rosemary wondered what her daughter's real state of mind and body might be. It was a relief that the operation was over, but the threat remained.

Jane had a single room in the small, modern hospital, and Rosemary found her the next day sitting up bright-eyed and cheerful. The pain was masked by her relief that the sinister lump was gone. In the days that followed she tried not to worry about the future. She complained only of the pain. Lymph glands drain fluid from the body, and nobody had warned her that, when this gland was removed from her groin, her right leg would become swollen and heavy with liquid. It was many days before an understanding nurse raised the foot of the bed for her, easing the pressure.

There were supposed to be only two visitors at a time in her room, but Jane often presided over a group of five or six friends clustered round the bed. The long visiting hours and the companionship of the nurses helped to keep her worries at bay, but there were many times when she was alone. She wrote in her diary:

'I don't want to have cancer. I don't want pain and I don't want to die for a long time. . . . The awful thing is not knowing even if they've dealt with this one, but . . . there seems to be a very high chance of others. And if I'm going to have to spend a large part of the rest of my life in pain and in hospital, I think I'd prefer to die quickly.

'The first birds have started to sing. Very beautiful. I think I'll just lie back and listen.'

Next day she wrote:

'I spent quite a lot of time yesterday wondering whether I would have the courage to kill myself if it looked as if the indefinite future was going to be spent in this way. And of course I came to no conclusion.'

Late in the evening of the tenth day the surgeon told Jane the bad news that the tumour had been malignant. All her fears had been confirmed. Rosemary was about to leave the hospital, but the ward sister called her back and said she didn't have to keep to the official visiting hours that evening. So she was able to comfort Jane and stay with her until she could cope. Sleeping pills would help her through the night.

Jane wrote: 'I'm not really sure what my reaction is. On the surface I'm very calm, very philosophical. I'm also aware that many people with cancer are cured completely. Also that very many do die.'

And the next day:

'Fear is always worst at night. Right now I feel awful . . . I'm waiting for the drugs, because I'm just scared I'll get the horrors if I try to sleep without them.'

A few days later, Rosemary was going through the daily routine of watering the plants and bulbs that stood on the long windowsill by the hospital bed, nipping off the dead blooms, when Jane said casually: 'By the way, Mum, I've found out the name of the cancer I've got. It's melanoma.'

Rosemary's hand froze.

Melanoma. The word had touched a chord in her memory. 'Melanomas can have your leg off in a week,' someone had once said. At the time it meant nothing to her. She was to find out that melanoma could be a killer, fast-moving and hard to treat. But it wasn't always fatal. And while it could be very painful, that was not always the case.

She phoned Victor and Richard on the other side of the Atlantic. In Boston, Richard called Joan at work. Her family had had experience of this deadly cancer. 'Joan,' he said, 'it's melanoma,' and put down the phone and wept.

Rosemary had promised to tell Jane the truth, but now she was hesitant. It wasn't easy to determine the precise truth. The right moment to reveal bad news has a habit of receding, and besides, there seemed to be so many views of Jane's chances. Every different opinion tended to increase the doubt and confusion. It was like appearing in court expecting a death sentence and discovering the judge didn't want to commit himself.

Behind Jane's back, we tried to get a clear medical prediction about the future, but without success. Richard was convinced Jane would receive more up-to-date treatment in America. Victor, with his usual thoroughness and persistence, began to investigate the possibilities of treatment in American hospitals. But Jane wanted to be near her friends. She showed no interest in leaving England, only in leaving the hospital.

After ten days she was discharged and referred to a specialist in a different London hospital for further tests. On the evening she came home, Richard phoned from Boston, wanting to know if she was aware of the danger.

'She realises it's serious,' said Rosemary cautiously, certain that Jane could hear her.

'But does she realise *how* serious?'

Rosemary lowered her voice slightly, but not enough to make Jane think she didn't want her to hear. 'I don't know.' It was a pretty ambiguous answer, the best she could do.

'Have you told her there's a strong probability she might die?' Richard burst out.

'Not exactly . . .'

'She ought to be told,' Richard said emphatically. 'She'd want to know.' He sounded sure, positive. 'Shall I tell her?'

'No.' *Not now*, Rosemary thought, but merely said: 'Jane's home from the hospital, but it'll take her a while to get to the phone, she's still weak.' Richard would surely pick up the message that her first night out of hospital wasn't the time to make such a disclosure. She was exhausted but seemed happy. Let her enjoy it, at least for a short time. Damn the future. After all, Rosemary consoled herself, none of the physicians Victor and Richard consulted had even seen Jane – and Jane's doctors didn't speak of death. When Richard spoke directly to Jane on the phone, he talked of other things.

Hope was our official attitude. Rosemary's friends supported her attempts to keep Jane's spirits up, but it was clear that at times she felt very alone, and Victor and Richard weren't yet free to come over.

A few nights before Jane's return from hospital, Teresa had phoned from America and asked simply, 'Do you want me to come?' Teresa was almost a daughter to Rosemary, almost a sister to Jane. She was Rosemary's most successful pottery student, now established in her own right in America. Her presence would help enormously, but Rosemary felt she couldn't ask Teresa to drop everything and leave her husband, her own work. 'It's all right, really,' she told her. 'I can cope.'

But as soon as Teresa rang off, Rosemary wished she'd said, 'Yes, please come.' She badly needed a full-time helper, with no other commitments, to share the burden.

Then the phone rang again. Rosemary answered unwillingly, dreading yet another family call, more pressure to take Jane to America for treatment there.

'Rosemary? Teresa here. I'm flying on Wednesday. Don't bother to meet me, I'll make my own way . . .'

Chapter 2

Teresa's arrival brought new vitality into the house. She came with special recipes for nourishing, health-giving foods to rebuild her friend's resources, so sadly depleted by three weeks of a hospital diet not intended for vegetarians. Jane had been scornful of the food given her: 'Cheese, tomato and *white* bread with a lettuce leaf one day. Tomato, cheese and two lettuce leaves the next. . . .' Teresa fed her protein the way she liked it, tasty and sustaining, and also brought more energy into the struggle to keep up her spirits.

To deal with her worst enemy – fear – Jane needed company, she needed distraction, she needed hope. She tried to fight off her fear by learning about melanoma, but this wasn't easy to do. People were reluctant to give her the information she sought. Friends promised books on cancer and mysteriously failed to deliver them. The statistics on the mortality rates for melanoma which she constantly requested were never provided. Rosemary couldn't tell her the stark facts and wouldn't let anyone in the family do it. Jane had friends who were nurses, and they came and spoke to her for hours about cancer in general and melanoma in particular, but Rosemary never learned what was said except that they talked about the various kinds of therapy. That much Rosemary knew from what Jane told her, yet her daughter didn't share everything. Rosemary was very afraid that she would learn the truth about melanoma – the terrible truth.

Jane tried to be philosophical. She spoke of accepting whatever came without a fight. If another tumour grew – 'and I suppose deep down, as a natural pessimist, I'm ready for the worst' – maybe she would live what was left of her life without any further operations or treatments.

Rosemary promised that if that was what she wanted, they would go away together and find a quiet, beautiful place to live, by the sea, perhaps. Or a special place for people with cancer she'd read about. 'It's not a hospital or a nursing home, it's more like a real home,' Rosemary recalled. 'The article said they treated everyone like people, not just patients, and looked after them with love and compassion. Shall I try to find out a bit more?'

'Yes . . .' Jane sounded doubtful. 'It may be a religious place. They wouldn't like a God-less type like me there. Even if they did take me, I don't know that I'd want to be in that sort of atmosphere. I wouldn't fit in. I'd feel bad about being there just because I needed to be and not because I had the same values.'

Nevertheless, Rosemary made enquiries and found out about St. Christopher's Hospice, designed to care for the terminally ill. It was indeed 'religious', but not in the sense Jane suspected. Although Dr. Cicely Saunders, who had founded St. Christopher's and thereby launched the modern hospice movement, was a committed Christian, she did not require her patients to be religious. The hospice was on the outskirts of London, set among green lawns which Jane would find a welcome sight. But would she qualify for admission?

Patients who still have a reasonable hope of being cured do not usually go to a hospice, whose aim is to improve the quality of their life for the last weeks or months. An individual is admitted for the control of distressing symptoms or because the family is unable to cope, or to give relatives a rest. Of those taken in, more than two-thirds are suffering unrelieved pain. A hospice prefers not to admit a patient only for the last few hours of life, for the last day or two, because so much less can be accomplished in so short a time. Generally a hospice would seek to assure itself that the prognosis promises the patient enough time to let the patient benefit from its special kind of help, to make it possible for her to live as fully as her physical condition allows. For this she must first be made comfortable, and helped to remain clear-headed, so that she may appreciate the love and care of family, friends, and the staff, reciprocate their feelings, and not imagine herself to be unwanted and abandoned, as happens to so many patients when those around them decide nothing more can be done. At St. Christopher's, Rosemary learned, there was always something that could be done for the patient, right to the very end. If the first attempt to relieve the pain and ease the discomfort didn't work, other approaches would be tried until the right one was found. All the time the patient would know that she mattered as a human being. As Cicely Saunders summed it up, 'You matter because you are you. You matter to the last moment of your life, and we will do all we can not only to help you die peacefully, but also to live until you die.'

Rosemary discussed what she had learned about St. Christopher's with Teresa, who waited for the right moment to broach the subject with Jane. But when Teresa suggested that they should all go to the hospice to give it the once over, Jane was no longer interested. By then she had decided not to give in, but to fight. She would insist that 'they' give her every possible treatment to drive back the cancer. She wanted to live.

Yet so much depended on her mood. There were times when she thought of death, the kind of planned death she had pondered over to her diary at the time of the second operation. Now she was quite willing to speak openly to Rosemary about it, as if to prepare her and ask her help. 'If I'm going to keep growing lumps and having them cut off – well, I don't know that I want to go on having that kind of life. I think I might just get out.'

Rosemary picked up her meaning immediately. She'd been thinking along the same lines, wondering whether such a life would be worth living. She too decided it was time to speak plainly.

'You know, Jane, if you really want to kill yourself, I'll help you as much as I can. You can be sure of that.'

'Thanks, Mum.' Jane smiled wanly.

'You remember my potter friend, Frances?' Rosemary went on. 'She nearly did it by mistake – at least, she said it was a mistake. She took sleeping pills and then carried a bottle of booze to bed with her in case they didn't work. It

29

would have been lethal if she hadn't been found in time. She said it was delicious.'

'There's only one snag.' Jane giggled. 'I don't like alcohol. So I'm not likely to do it.'

The conversation lingered in Rosemary's mind. Had her promise of help been too facile? How could one be sure that Jane really wanted to commit suicide, however ill and pain-ridden she became? Might there not be down-days followed immediately by up-days? Suppose she had hung on a little longer and a cure was discovered? Wasn't the taking of life – any life – a terrible thing? Rosemary also wondered if her offer of 'help' to Jane wouldn't be in itself a form of pressure, a hidden suggestion that they would all be much better off without her. Since her illness, Jane had often expressed concern that she was 'mucking up' Rosemary's life. And what would the rest of the family think about it?

Early one morning Rosemary was awakened by a phone call from Victor, his voice made unfamiliar by the distance, high and strained.

'Have you thought any more about her coming to America? There could be a lot of advantages here.'

'She's much too ill to cross the Atlantic,' Rosemary said wearily, pulling her nightgown closer around her for warmth. 'I told you, she's very weak. Her leg is still swollen. She won't even come to the park in the car.'

Victor said urgently: 'Listen, Rosemary, I've been talking to some of the world's top cancer experts. They're making a lot of progress in treating cancer here. They'll take her in at the National Cancer Institute . . .'

'I've told you she's much too weak . . .'

'They're doing a lot of work on melanoma. They'll take her as a research patient. They'll give her all the latest – '

'My God, *research?*' Nobody, Rosemary swore silently to herself, would use Jane for experiments, for testing untried drugs. 'What would that mean, for God's sake?'

'They really are some of the best doctors in the States.' Now he was trying to placate her, his voice gentle. 'They'd look after her well and she'd have a better chance.'

'I keep telling you, she can't walk properly yet, much less hop in and out of airplanes. She doesn't *want* to come,' she almost shouted. 'She wants to be near her friends.'

'Are you all right?'

Suddenly Rosemary felt exhausted, limp. 'I'm all right,' she murmured. 'Goodbye,' and she hung up on him. She knew that it was time for Victor to come to England. Jane was in for a terrible experience: pain, operations, treatments. The pain would probably change and destroy her. Victor should see her as she was now, strong – at least most of the time – determined, and full of humour. She could still turn her despair into a joke. Victor ought to talk with her at leisure and clear up their past differences, get to know her better, while there was still time.

After Jane had breakfasted and was enjoying the first cigarette of the day, Rosemary asked her: 'What do you think about Dad coming over? I feel he's missing a lot by not being here now.'

'Wouldn't it be easier if he didn't?' Jane responded. 'Dad always makes such a crisis over everything and we've got quite enough crisis already.' She lit up another cigarette. 'Let's wait and see what happens when I visit the doctor next week.'

She was quiet for a long time. Then she said sadly: 'They told me that if melanoma "crosses your womb" – whatever that means – you shouldn't have a baby for at least ten years. Even if I do make it that long, I'll be getting a bit old. It'd be risky. Did you know the incidence of brain-damaged or retarded kids gets much higher when you're near forty? I'd have liked to have had kids.'

She asked Rosemary to make a cup of coffee. Then, as soon as her mother was out of the room, she turned to Teresa. 'Its OK now, but suppose I get much worse and have a lot of pain? I really can't take pain well. I've been storing up pills, just in case. Olivia had a whole bottle, but if I ask her for them she'd feel involved if I took them. I don't think I should put that on her.' (Olivia was the friend in whose house they were staying.)

'Have you talked about it to Rosemary?'

'We did a bit. But I think she'd feel guilty if I involved her. If I do myself in, I'll do it on my own.'

Teresa said nothing about this conversation to Rosemary,

who, unaware of Jane's real feelings, brought up the subject again a few days later. 'I told you I'd help you if you wanted to commit suicide, Jane. I've thought about it a lot since – of course I'll help you. But we'll both have to be really sure that you mean it. Things can change from day to day. And Dad and Richard ought to know . . . they have a right to be part of such a big thing.' Jane listened carefully but didn't reply. 'Besides,' Rosemary tried to make a joke of it, 'they might think I'd done you in because I couldn't take it!'

Later Rosemary was to regret that conversation. She wished she hadn't seemed to renege on a promise, a matter of trust between them.

Jane was home for just over a week before she saw the specialist. He said she should enter a London hospital for further tests.

She wrote in her diary of the help and support she was getting, but added: 'Despite all this I feel totally alone. It is good to have people around and I know quite a few are really affected by the whole business. It reminds them of their own mortality and of humanity's abysmal ignorance of what cancer is, and of course they are aware it isn't much fun for me.

'The ignorance is one of the worst things. And it isn't just that doctors are so bad at telling one what they are doing and why, and what is likely to happen. But also that so little is actually known and there is so much difference of opinion among the specialists.'

This time Jane was in hospital for ten days. Every possible area of her body was tested for the presence of cancer, and every test came up with the same result: negative. This should have been cause for rejoicing, but she still had the brain scan to experience. At one time frequent attacks of dizziness made her think that the cancer had spread to her brain, and she was very frightened. 'The possibility of a brain tumour is too awful to contemplate,' she wrote. 'I know that it's just that they're doing everything to rule things out. But this has upset me more than anything. I'm simply terrified. . . .' When this test also proved negative, she allowed herself a tempered sense of relief. 'But just because the X-rays are clear doesn't mean there is nothing there.'

It was the bone marrow test she found most painful and objectionable. They should have prepared her, she said crossly. They'd told her it might be 'a bit uncomfortable,' but it was actually much worse than that – 'absolutely disgusting.'

She wasn't in much pain, but her diary revealed the anguish she was experiencing: 'It is frightening to be so weak. One is so used to a more or less normally functioning body that it takes both physical and emotional adjusting to a situation in which walking is difficult and something of an ordeal. Then there is the feeling of envy – often near jealousy – of those who are able to walk, run, move with ease and simply keep going all day.

'At times I've felt so ill it's an effort to move at all. And it's then that I really do feel there is something seriously wrong with me. Other times I don't feel too bad and wonder whether it's my mind or body that holds the weakness. When I do feel ill I have very little interest in cancer or in anything else. Also I get very scared of being alone and getting the horrors. But I do only seem to break down when there's someone around to help.

'I've just realised something that is probably very evident. That is that there are two types of fear. The first is the irrational kind, what I call the "horrors", when all I can think of is the cancer probably in my body eating away at the healthy parts and taking over. And the best way to cope with this is by trying to analyse what it is I'm scared of. Pain, or death, or uncertainty, or the effect on my life and psyche. And these are fears which can be coped with. The "horrors" are not rational and I cannot banish them by trying to concentrate on something else, but I can cope with them by trying to translate them into the second kind – into other, manageable fears.'

Jane was able to come home for the weekend, but the return on Sunday night was like escorting her back to some gruesome kind of boarding school. She had to be taken to the hospital like a child – a child unable to manage the journey alone. She needed an arm to lean on while walking, someone to carry her bag, someone to pay the cab driver quickly so she didn't have to be on her feet longer than was necessary to walk to the busy, anonymous ward.

When Jane was with Teresa and Rosemary, they were all a family; but when she was in the hospital, Teresa and Rosemary were strongly aware of their isolation, separated not only from Jane but from the everyday world. Nothing could be planned or taken for granted. They fought off their despair, struggling to behave as if life were still the same, but always aware how fragile the pretence was. Friends did their best to give support – there was always someone to offer strength and practical help when needed.

One evening Rosemary was coming home from visiting Jane alone, stale from the long hospital hours and thinking of how little could be done for her daughter. She remembered how Jane had always valued solitude, and now she was trapped in a crowded ward. Rosemary was seized by a violent desire to cut and run, to escape. A cab rounded the corner and she wanted to jump in, drive to the airport, get on a plane, and fly – where? There was nowhere to go. Jane needed her. This was not the time to give in to despair. And there was some good news.

None of the other hospital tests showed the slightest trace of any more tumours in Jane's body. It was settled that she could leave; the next step was for the doctors to decide what preventive treatment she should have. Our hopes revived again.

The evening before Jane was due to come out of the hospital, Teresa and Rosemary went to a play in London to celebrate. It was Jane's idea. But they returned home to find that Jane had been trying to reach them. She had just been examined by the doctor she liked and trusted most. Dr. Byrd was an elegant woman who had always been most patient and understanding in answering Jane's many questions about her illness. Jane used to compile lists before each of her visits. Sometimes she would still be busy writing when the doctor arrived. Dr. Byrd hadn't said much, but later a nurse brought a message telling Jane to ask her mother to come to the hospital the next day. The surgeon wanted to see them both together. The unexpectedness of this request made Jane very anxious. She wanted consolation from Rosemary and Teresa, but they, too, were fearful. Was the run of good luck already over?

The surgeon was grave and direct.

During the routine examination another lump had been noticed at a higher location in Jane's body. It would have to be removed as soon as a bed was free. Jane and Rosemary exchanged hopeless looks: a third operation. First the black spot on the foot, then the lymphatic gland in the groin, and now a tumour on the wall of her stomach. It seemed like a deadly progression.

Jane kept her composure until she was back in the ward. Then she was suddenly crying out loud, the tears streaming down her face. One of the nurses appeared with surprising speed, carrying a tray with a syringe.

'I'm all right. I don't want anything,' Jane protested quickly. She tried to control herself, sitting up on the bed and feeling blindly for her clothes, her eyes still blurred with tears. 'Let's get the hell out of here.'

Now a doctor appeared behind the nurse. 'Tell them all to go away.' Jane sounded angry, and the doctor and nurse hesitated.

Rosemary tried to reassure them. 'She's all right now, thank you.'

Jane regained control and they quickly left the hospital. But it was a slow crawl home by cab through the rush-hour traffic. Jane caught glimpses of the daffodils massed under the trees in a park – it was the middle of March and there were flowers everywhere.

Meanwhile, Victor had learned that Britain and the United States share the results of cancer research. Jane would get equally up-to-date treatment in either country, so the pressure on Rosemary to persuade Jane to go to America was off. No one could be sure of Jane's future, the family could make no definite plans. They must live from hour to hour, day to day, coping with the continuous anxiety and uncertainty as best they could.

Jane stayed in bed, read a lot, wrote letters and telephoned and entertained her friends. These visits helped by giving her a life of her own, keeping her from feeling too much the helpless invalid. It wasn't all gloom. She had stories to tell us, news and jokes from visitors.

'I don't know why they come,' she said one day. 'I seem to

spend most of the time talking about cancer, it must get pretty dull. I hope to goodness nobody gets sick of me and stops coming.'

'I'm certain they get pleasure from being with you,' Rosemary assured her. 'It's a mutual thing. People might come once or twice out of pity or sympathy, but they'd soon stop if they didn't enjoy talking to you.'

Jane burst suddenly into a happy laugh. 'Michael says I'm the worst advertisement for health foods he's ever met!'

Michael had been Jane's first love in her Sussex University days. The two years they spent together in Brighton, the vacations they had taken in Europe and the United States, proved to be the great adventure of their lives. They each explored the other's personality to new depths and were astonished at the treasures they found. Jane stimulated Michael's political awakening and guided his emergence from a sheltered middle-class background until he came to exceed her zeal for left-wing causes. But Jane's interests were turning to the women's movement. They had been so absorbed in each other, so close, that at times it seemed as if she hardly had a life of her own, and this scared her. She began to pull back. This in turn caused tensions which neither of them knew how to handle, until she decided to make a clean break, to free herself from this new dependence.

Michael tried to understand her need for 'space', as they termed it in their long, anguished, deeply analytical discussions of the relationship, but he didn't think it called for such a drastic step. Jane, however, was not to be talked out of her decision. Michael could only vow to himself that he would always be there when she needed him. In the years that followed they were to come together again several times when Jane's loneliness got the better of her determination to protect her independence. Now, as her illness grew, he returned once more to give her the support she craved, and a new love began to develop between them, hesitant, uncertain of the future, but very important to Jane at this crisis in her life.

Chapter 3

One day a faith healer arrived to see Jane. She had been urged by a friend of Rosemary, who was prepared to try anything. Mrs. Claire was marvellous, Rosemary was told. She didn't always cure, but she often helped sick people with the problems of adjusting to illness.

'Why is this woman coming?' Jane asked bitterly that morning. 'I won't see her. I don't want any faith healers. What good can she do?'

Rosemary reminded her calmly that she'd agreed earlier the visit wouldn't do any harm and might be interesting. 'She thinks she can help you. She's driving a long way to get here. But if you really don't want her to come into your room, I'll just give her tea and she can go.'

Jane gave way grudgingly. 'I suppose she'll have to come in once she's here.'

Mrs. Claire was a small, round woman with soft, grey eyes and grey curls framing her face. She puffed up the stairs to Jane's room with great dignity. She had an air of authority combined with a certain motherliness. The fact that Victor would have disapproved so completely of the visit gave Rosemary a mild thrill.

Jane had settled down and politely began to play the hostess. The faith healer asked for a bowl of hot water. She then pulled back the bedcover and showed no surprise that Jane, who disliked wearing nightclothes, was naked. Mrs. Claire dipped her hands in the hot water and shook them violently, scattering drops in a wide area around Jane. Then she drew her wet hands slowly over the naked body, pressing hard into the flesh as if forcing the illness down, from shoulder to fingertip, from hip to toe. After each sweep, she would shake her arms from the elbows, as if to rid them of the evil extracted by her movements.

At the end, Mrs. Claire said: 'Now you will sleep. Tomorrow you will feel better.' She pulled the bedclothes up over Jane's still body and quietly left the room.

Downstairs in the hall she said to Rosemary: 'She is very, very sick. But I'm prepared to treat her. Can she stop all the hospital treatments?'

Her offer was obviously serious and sincere. Rosemary responded hesitantly. 'I'll talk about it with her . . . I'll call you. Thank you very much for coming.' She felt in her purse. 'I'd like . . .'

'Just my expenses for the journey, dear,' said Mrs. Claire emphatically. 'Nothing more. It wouldn't be right. And whatever you decide to do, I will be thinking about Jane. My friends will be thinking of her, too.'

Rosemary tiptoed upstairs to find Jane wide-awake. 'Mrs. Claire told me she could cure me if I really believed.' Jane sounded matter-of-fact. 'But I know I couldn't be sure – it didn't seem possible. I couldn't risk it.'

Much later she told her mother that it was then, after the faith healer had left, that she'd known she was soon going to die. She had started to fall asleep, but was filled with a deep sense of fear and despair and realised there was no hope.

A short time after Mrs. Claire's visit, Rosemary was woken in the night by a cry of anguish. Jane was out of bed, flexing her leg. 'Such a horrible pain in my side – I must have been lying wrong,' she muttered.

It was at that moment that Rosemary in turn realised Jane was going to die. The knowledge remained with her: an inner certainty and a basic acceptance of the inevitable loss. Yet whenever the disease took another turn or there was a false alarm, the sense of anguish Rosemary felt would increase to crisis pitch. Was that another mole growing? Another lump? Every step in Jane's illness, inevitable as we suspected it to be, was nevertheless an unexpected blow, and she had to muster new resources to overcome it. Teresa and Jane fought too, each in her own way. The fear was always there between the three of us – silent, something to be pushed back, mastered. We didn't talk much about this. Most of the time our efforts to make life as pleasant as possible for each other succeeded.

We had acquired a new ally in Michael, whose visits gave Jane a different kind of reassurance. He refused to admit even to himself the seriousness of Jane's condition, and whenever she grew depressed he worked hard to instil in her a fresh determination to fight her illness. He used their old love as the weapon with which to ward off the threat to her. He knew best how to be close to her, as close as any two human beings can be, and he burrowed into their joint memory of the Brighton years to dig out the past. Sometimes it was as simple as using the old expressions whose meaning only the two of them knew: not just the endearments but also the words that had acquired a special significance denoting a shared experience and a common view of other people, of events they had lived through, and of life itself. At other times it could be as delicate as bringing to the surface detailed recollections of old times when there had been friction as well as harmony between them. His attempt to reactivate their old relationship involved risks for both.

Michael held Jane's hand, kissed her, embraced her gently to avoid hurting her. Physical contact had been important to them then, and now Michael made deliberate use of it to tell her, more emphatically than words could, 'You're still Jane.' She had not said that this was the kind of reassurance she wanted, not in so many words, but perhaps she had conveyed her need for it when she complained of her swollen leg, of the ugly scar left by her operation.

Putting his arm around her, Michael tried to persuade Jane to get out of bed, helped her to walk down the stairs, then urged her softly to go up again. He explained to her why this was important, how it would contribute to her recovery, speed it up. 'I know it hurts, but you've got to do it.' And she did.

Jane responded emotionally, too, opening up to Michael in a way she had not done since the Brighton days. 'Apart from Mum and Teresa,' she wrote in her diary, 'the person who has helped me most and to whom I've felt closest is Michael. I have felt very near to him physically and emotionally. The few times we've been alone I've felt that we really do belong together and that part of me – a very suppressed part – has been missing him since we split up.'

But did she have the right to fall in love all over again, and to draw Michael in with her? She wrote of the 'danger' of becoming too involved with him and of what this might lead to. 'I have just used the word "danger". Why? Is it because I am scared of becoming too dependent? Of hurting him? Of him not caring for me?'

Or was it because she knew how uncertain the future was? 'Is it because this whole cancer business has made me more vulnerable, more in need of people, and when I sense him caring for me, is it not purely for me, but for me in my present situation?' Michael himself, when he later recalled these days, did not find it easy to disentangle his motives. He and Jane had come closer to each other again shortly before she left for Greece. The process of mutual rediscovery had fascinated them, and both regretted that they had kept their distance for so long; but they remained deliberately casual about it. 'If I wasn't going abroad,' Jane wrote at the time, 'I'd probably be tempted into having a full-blown affair with him.' So Michael was the first person she phoned the day she came back from Greece and got the bad news from Dr. Sullivan.

Now, after three weeks with us, Teresa had to go back to America. She would have given anything to put her arms round our daughter and say simply: 'Jane, you're going to die, let's talk about it.' It was only in deference to Rosemary that she said nothing. Ironically, Jane's mother didn't know what Teresa was thinking. Rosemary believed that she and Teresa had understood each other perfectly, that they had agreed not to tell Jane how slight her chances were. In fact Rosemary was deceiving herself, because that was what she wanted to believe. Teresa had agreed to no such thing.

Richard and Joan had arranged to fly over from Boston to take Teresa's place, and Rosemary was fearful that they might just burst in, tired and strained, and tell Jane the truth outright. Teresa agreed to meet them at the airport and discuss this with them. 'When they go back, I think Victor should come. You shouldn't be alone,' she added.

The next morning Teresa met Richard and Joan at the London air terminal and took them to a café to talk. Richard was tired and strained. 'I think Mum's hiding her head in the sand and not facing up to reality. She won't admit to herself that Jane's going to die and she won't let any of us tell her. That's wrong.'

'Rosemary feels we shouldn't tell her there's no hope,' Teresa pointed out. 'The doctors agree. But whatever happens, it's Rosemary who will have to deal with the situation as it develops. You'll be back in Boston, Richard. I think Rosemary should handle it as she needs to and we should support her.'

'If Jane knew she hadn't long to live she could choose what she wanted to do with the time she has left.'

'There's not much she can do at the moment,' Teresa said. 'Just lie in bed and wait for the next operation.'

Joan spoke up: 'Suppose she'd rather not have this operation?'

'She knows that if she doesn't have it, she'll die,' Teresa answered. 'She wants any treatment she can get. She got real mad when one of the doctors waved chemotherapy aside and said it was of no positive value for her.'

But, Joan persisted, would Jane still feel the same if she knew how little chance she had of recovering? Teresa had no reply. All she could say was, 'She keeps pressing for statistics, and we just hedge.'

Jane was delighted to see her brother again. She knew she could rely on him for help, both practical and emotional. She remembered how protective he'd been during their childhood. She looked up to him and admired him – most of the time, anyway. We had tried to bring both children up to have an equal share of whatever was available: schooling, holidays, pocket money, treats. But things aren't always so easy. The older child is nearly always ahead, stronger, more experienced. Inevitably, Richard took command when they were little – a fact that Jane sometimes resented but usually came to accept. In her teens, Richard encouraged Jane's attempts to find her own life style, away from the family pattern. He was ready with advice and offers of practical help when she needed it. They had been close in their childhood, but for several years since he had left England to go to Harvard they had seen little of each other, only meeting for brief periods. Now she wrote in her diary: 'It doesn't feel as if it's been a long time since we saw each other and I find I like him a great deal as a person.'

There had been a time, before their teens, when the relationship between Richard and Jane was in bad shape. They fought continually, each playing on the other's weaknesses until the whole family grew strained and irritable. Then we bought a boat and spent our weekends aboard. Our lives were transformed. Every voyage became an adventure. Arguments continued, but were more often concerned with the processes of learning new skills: sailing, rowing, lighting camp fires and mastering the problems of outdoor cooking. Their early relationship, trusting on her part, protective on his, was basically restored. They grew up, became self-reliant, and as they advanced into their teens learned to act in more adult ways. Soon boyfriends and girlfriends appeared on the scene, but by that time Richard had gone on an English-Speaking Union scholarship to America. Jane saw him only during the vacations, either in England or in the United States, usually in the company of his current girl-friend. Now, on meeting Joan for the first time, she wrote: 'Joan is extremely nice, but I feel we're not totally at ease with each other and it may be my fault. Joan obviously means far, far more to him than anyone else has done and I am glad for them both and think they are good for each other. But maybe a part of me wants Richard for myself.'

As it turned out, Jane quickly developed a good relationship with her brother's fiancée. Joan, who had been a para-medic, was both knowledgeable and direct, and Jane could see she was eager to help in every way she could.

Jane wanted to know everything Joan and Richard could tell her about melanoma. She apparently sensed that she was being kept outside the knowledge the rest of the family shared. But she could communicate easily with Joan, and it was to her that she first put the question: 'Am I dying?'

Joan could only answer that it was impossible to know.

She thought Jane should share in the whole truth, but obeyed Rosemary's embargo. She herself had worked as a hospital volunteer when she was only twelve years old, and had often sat with the dying when the doctors and nurses had given up hope. In that hosital nobody was ever officially declared to be dying, but the messages of rejection were quickly picked up by the staff, and usually by the patients too.

Two days after their arrival was Jane's twenty-fifth birthday. She woke with a blinding headache, in a deep depression. She lay all day in a darkened room, unable to bear even a crack of light. The bedroom quickly filled with flowers and birthday presents as friends arrived, but Jane could neither talk to them nor look at their gifts. Michael, who had so often managed to cheer her up, was upset at his failure to do so this time. Nothing helped her until the end of the day, when Richard went in for yet another attempt to talk to his sister, to get her to voice her misery. Then she wept and felt better – well enough to invite us all to have supper in her room. Soon she was sitting up and laughing, cracking jokes.

But behind the scenes we were preparing for the third operation. We had rented a flat near the hospital. We were anxious that Jane's morale should be as high as possible and her stay in the hospital no worse than it had to be. The day before she went in, Richard recorded tapes of her favourite music. He planned to buy earphones for the tape recorder so she could listen to music without disturbing the other patients, but first he had to find out which earphones were the lightest, the most comfortable in bed, and the most dependable at conveying the best sound. The recorder and earphones would help Jane to escape from the noises of the hospital ward – she particularly hated the distorted, pervasive TV – and from unwanted conversations when she was feeling low.

The disagreement about how much of the truth Jane should be told kept surfacing. Rosemary admired Richard for his commitment to the truth, but she was still unsure whether Jane was ready for it.

As he recorded the music, Richard told his mother: 'Jane said if there's only a ten per cent chance of her surviving this, she'll give up. I've given her the impression it's roughly a one-in-three chance she'll recover, but of course it's much less. It's pretty hellish not being able to be straight with her.'

'I thought one in three was about right. Teresa rang a doctor friend and she gave us those figures,' Rosemary countered quickly.

'That was before we knew she had to have another operation. Now it's much lower.'

Rosemary felt cornered. 'I don't think statistics mean much. What is a statistic? When it's you or me, that's different from a number on a piece of paper. I'm sick of all this talk of statistics.'

Joan came into the room, taking care to shut the door behind her. 'I've been talking with Jane about mind over matter. I told her about the cancer research to determine whether sick people who were religious actually had a higher survival rate than atheists. The statistics showed that both deeply religious people and strong atheists had the same chance – it was the half-believers, the people who weren't sure, who had a lower survival rate.'

'How did she react?' Rosemary was aware that Joan was on Richard's side.

'She was terrifically pleased. It took a load off her mind. It was an awful feeling for her to have – that whenever she got depressed, she might be failing to keep herself alive.'

'We ought to be quite plain with her,' Richard said abruptly. 'We should just tell her.'

'There's another point, Rich.' It still seemed to Rosemary that death was probably far enough away for Jane to believe she had some life left to live. 'You know how depressed Jane can get and what a pain in the neck she can be. If we tell her she's finished and she goes right down, then nobody will want to be with her. What keeps her so balanced – and remember, she only collapses with us, she's usually bright and positive with others – is having so many friends visiting and holding the outside world open. If she sinks into withdrawal, they'll soon give up coming. Nobody will want to talk to someone who won't respond. She'll have a really miserable existence.'

'You could be right,' Richard conceded reluctantly.

Rosemary pressed her advantage. 'She gets so much happiness from the visits, the flowers, the phone calls. Just think, the alternative might be for her to lie silent and withdrawn in increasing pain while the illness gains ground. That's a pretty grim prospect for her – and for the rest of us, come to that. After all, Rich, it can be argued that we're all due to die one day. I might go under a bus tomorrow . . .'

'Mum,' said Richard impatiently, 'I think you're evading the issue when you talk like that.'

'That's enough for the moment.' Rosemary retreated to the door. 'Jane'll think we're talking about her – which we are. I'll take her up some coffee.'

End of argument – until the next round.

We tried to make sure Jane didn't feel she was isolated, but it wasn't easy. And we made mistakes.

'Rosemary,' Joan said later the same day, 'Do you realise – when you were talking in the hall yesterday – Jane could hear every word?'

'My God! What was I saying?'

'Nothing much, but she heard it all quite clearly. I thought you'd want to know.'

Rosemary tried to remember everything she'd said. Had there been anything that could have killed whatever hope Jane might have left? She had been relieved to learn that Teresa had talked with Jane about the future and Jane had seemed strangely matter-of-fact about her chances. 'I don't know what all this fuss is about,' she had said wryly. 'The worst thing that can happen is that I shall die.'

While the operation was in progress, Rosemary remembered that remark. We were aware how serious the situation was. The cancer was in the centre of Jane's body. It was possible she might die if things went wrong – we wondered if that would not be preferable to the succession of operations that seemed almost inevitable. We distracted ourselves as best we could until it was over and Richard could phone for news. He was told that Jane was doing well.

Yet this time her recovery was very slow. For days she lay virtually motionless, barely talking, eating almost nothing.

Richard, Joan, and Rosemary took turns sitting with her, but her friends were told not to come for a while.

The surgeon explained to Rosemary that he didn't think he had removed the whole of the cancer. He'd operated as far into her body as he could without endangering Jane's life, but the area beyond remained swollen. He believed the cancer was still there. 'What shall I tell her?' he asked kindly, and waited for Rosemary's reply. What could she say? It sounded like the death sentence for Jane.

'She'll have to know,' she murmured hesitantly. *I promised to tell her everything, but not now, not today.* Aloud she went on: 'She's so weak, let's wait until she's a bit stronger. Then we must tell her.'

The next day Jane was slightly better and there was some good news. A biopsy report showed there were no cancer cells remaining in the area after all. The swelling hadn't been caused by a tumour; it had been merely a reaction to the diseased area removed by the operation.

But in the following few days Jane didn't improve. There seemed to be little life left in her. The skin around her mouth was white, her eyes – when she opened them briefly – were un-focused and vague. She might have been in a void where the passage of time was meaningless. If she was experiencing any thoughts or feelings, nothing showed in her face.

Later, when she was alone, she was able to express herself in her diary in handwriting that was large, sprawling, uncertain:

'For most of the time I seem to have lost all sense of reality. I think I need a shrink or something. Most of the time I feel so ill that it doesn't matter. . . . I certainly can't relate much to anyone on the ward. The women are good-hearted enough and the one next to me is very concerned that I'm not eating enough. But the doctors and nurses don't give a shit. . . . It's incredibly difficult to write straight and I have at last found a tiny corner of reality. It certainly isn't adequate though.'

Rosemary was close to giving up all hope when suddenly there was a dramatic change in Jane's condition. She was able to sit up in bed and there was colour in her cheeks. The cause of this seeming miracle was a blood transfusion.

Jane had always been squeamish at the sight of blood. Now she had to put up with a whole plastic bagful of it, menacing, suspended over her head, filled with the red plasma that was a sickening reminder of the seriousness of her condition. The vertical metal stand looked firm enough, but the horizontal bracket which extended from it, and from which the bag was suspended, was designed to slide up and down as necessary and to be adjusted at varying heights. To Jane, with her aversion to this gibbet, the contraption looked anything but secure. She was attached to this monster by a thin red tube whose needle, taped into her vein, added to the irritation caused by the need to keep her wrist steady, fastened to a splint. The hated blood fed slowly, drip by drip, into her arm. She fretted about the tedious, continuous process, impatient for it to end, fearful that something might go wrong. During the night she began to worry that the bag wasn't held securely in place, and asked a nurse to check.

'It's perfectly all right,' said the nurse, after a glance at the blood transfusion unit.

Next day Jane told us how she had tried to hold the nurse's attention, longing for company to help her shake off the nightmare feeling of fear and isolation.

'I do feel very peculiar . . .' she had begun, but the cry for help went unrecognised.

'You must go to sleep now,' The nurse had said firmly. 'Everything is all right.'

In the middle of the night Jane was awakened from her deep, drugged sleep by a crash. The bar holding the drip feed bag had slid down the vertical stand and collapsed on her bed, dislodging the tube connecting her to the transfusion unit. The blood burst out, spattering all around, bright red on the white sheets, spreading over Jane herself as she recoiled in terror. The more she fidgeted, the bloodier she got. The liquid rapidly coagulated, sticking to her inexorably, making her look like a casualty. With Jane's particular fear of blood, the incident was a living nightmare, but by the time we arrived in the morning she had been cleaned up and had even managed to get more sleep. Only her indignation remained as she described the scene and spoke angrily of the nurse's off-hand attitude. Her resentment was greater than her fear. To her relief, no more transfusions were necessary.

But she was often in severe pain. When Rosemary pointed this out to the surgeon, he turned angrily to the house doctor. 'Why is this girl suffering? She should not have to be in pain!'

Rosemary saw one of the younger nurses in the corridor near tears. 'It's always the same,' the nurse half-shouted over her shoulder. 'The patients don't tell us what's wrong, then they complain and we get into trouble.'

Jane was not given additional medicine for many hours. The nurses said they had to wait for specific authority. When the doses were increased, she still complained of the pain. Rosemary told Richard that the house doctor, after being criticised by the surgeon, seemed to imply that Jane was playing up. 'I told him she always made a fuss when she was ill. Then I felt terribly disloyal. She really is suffering.'

'Jane never invented symptoms,' Richard said indignantly, 'and she's not making things up now.'

'I told him she'd been brave until the pain got bad. He just replied: "Ah yes, pain . . ." '

Later it was found that Jane was particularly resistant to drugs and needed heavier doses than many people. But she was now making steady progress, and friends could visit again. Sometimes the cancer ward had almost the atmosphere of a social club. Watching Jane with her friends and the other patients, we began to hope once more.

One afternoon she was enjoying a forbidden cigarette when there was a roar from the far corner of the ward.

'She's smoking again!' a little old woman shouted from her bed, frantic with fury and fear. 'She'll blow us all up! It's disgusting, absolutely disgusting. You ought to be ashamed of yourself!'

'How can it possibly blow anyone up?' Jane asked the world at large above the continuing mutter from the distant corner. 'What nonsense!'

The ward sister appeared. 'Jane,' she said, in a tone that was polite but firm, 'it really is dangerous. There are oxygen cylinders in here, and they might explode. You must go into the corridor if you want to smoke.'

Jane was not ready to leave her bed, so she put out the cigarette without argument. But she began to grumble when the ward sister was out of earshot, and the old woman muttered in her corner. The rest of the ward, mostly sympathetic to Jane because of her youth and serious illness, maintained a neutral silence.

Later, the ward sister spoke to Rosemary in her office. 'Jane really must make an effort to get out of bed and move around,' she said. 'She may have many months of lying in bed in the future. She should get up now, while she can.'

Rosemary argued that her daughter was very weak, that she wasn't pretending about the pain, and that so far the disease had moved more rapidly than they'd been led to expect.

The ward sister looked sympathetic, but still insisted that Jane should get up. It would be good for her body to be moving. She also spoke to Richard and Joan, who proved to be more realistic and less protective.

That evening Richard gave Jane a blunt lecture on the need to get out of bed. Jane listened, wept, protested, and eventually lost her temper. Richard persisted, but he went home worried that he had overdone it. Maybe Jane herself really knew what was best for her.

The ward sister was right. When we arrived the next day Jane was already out of bed, cheerful and hopeful. Michael also came that day. He was able to persuade her to sit in a wheelchair, and he pushed her into the corridor where she could smoke. Having only recently recovered from an appendectomy, he could relate to Jane's weakness and lack of confidence. He worked hard to steer her away from the preoccupation with illness that he felt was pulling her down, away from life. He urged her to leave the cancer ward and take the lift down to the hospital shop. At last she summoned up the courage to make the journey and they smoked a ceremonial cigarette together, four floors down, by the entrance to the hospital. Then Michael, still weak from his own operation, supported her back to bed.

We allowed ourselves to hope that Jane was in remission. There were no obvious new sources of cancer in her body, and although she was still ill, her pain and weakness might have been the result of the operation. Now the doctors saw it as their job to prevent the recurrence of cancer, to kill off any diseased cells that might still remain in her body before they had a chance to multiply and grow into tumours. This, they explained, could be done by chemotherapy, a treatment which had shown an increasing rate of success over the years as new research continued to produce more effective drugs. The drugs would be introduced into Jane's bloodstream by injection, and would travel around her body until they encountered a cancer cell. Then they would attack it, poison it, and kill it.

Jane was well aware that chemotherapy could have unpleasant side effects. She had seen women who had lost all their hair: one walked around the ward with a kerchief round her head; another wore a wig by courtesy of the National Health Service. Jane dreaded losing her hair, but she knew it did not happen in every case and she was prepared to risk it. Chemotherapy sometimes causes loss of hair because the drugs, to be effective, have to attack the most rapidly growing cells. Not all of these are cancer cells. The cells in the scalp grow very quickly, and some of the drugs, being unable to discriminate, attack them too. Other side effects can take the form of nausea, vomiting, diarrhoea. But these vary from person to person, depending on the combination of drugs chosen for each case and on the different reactions to them.

Jane's course of chemotherapy began with one injection a day for a week. Then she was to have a three-week rest, followed by other doses – one every month for about a year – until all the stray cancer cells in her body had been hunted down and killed.

Not long ago Rosemary had thought Jane was on the point of dying. Now they were starting on treatment that could last a year. Tomorrow, the picture could change again. Nothing seemed final, neither hope nor despair. Victor still put off flying from Washington. He had become optimistic. Even if Jane's chance of survival was only one in five – as he gathered from one set of statistics – he persisted in believing she would be lucky. He had always been lucky himself, especially during World War II when his life had been in danger several times.

When Rosemary urged him on the phone to lose no more

time in flying over, Victor repeated his old argument. If he came now, Jane would be bound to jump to the conclusion that he had returned because she was dying. 'Do we want her to think that?'

'I need you and Jane needs you,' Rosemary persisted. 'You must come now.'

He seemed not to have heard. 'Of course,' he said soothingly. 'When you want me, just tell me. I'll get on the next plane.'

'I'm telling you to come *now*, so that we can all talk together before Richard and Joan have to go back.' Her voice was high and strained, and she spoke slowly, with insulting clarity.

There was a short silence, then Victor said quietly: 'I'll come on Wednesday.'

When Jane was told her father was coming, she asked Joan: 'Is it because I'm getting worse?' Joan's answer was matter-of-fact. 'You know that Richard and I must go back soon. Your father wants to be with your mother and you.' Jane asked no more questions.

On the first day of the chemotherapy, Rosemary went to the hospital hoping that Jane would be one of the lucky ones and suffer few, if any, side effects. Her bed was empty. One of the other patients spoke to Rosemary. 'She's in the bathroom. Poor Jane. She's been terribly sick.' People murmured in sympathy.

The bathroom door was open. Rosemary slipped in, shutting the door behind her.

'Oh, Mum,' Jane wailed. 'I've been sick twelve times. I feel so awful!'

She was vomiting violently and continually, and struggling simultaneously with diarrhoea. When she was finally helped back to bed, she sank back and lay still, only to be racked over and over again by vomiting. The ward sister talked to her kindly, telling her it would soon be over. 'Every day it will get easier as your system gets adjusted to the treatment. You *will* feel better tomorrow, Jane. In the meantime we'll give you an anti-emetic injection which will stop the sickness.'

'I don't think I can go through with this,' Jane murmured

weakly, but we were determined not to let her give up, and finally persuaded her that she must continue with the treatment. Whenever she complained of nausea, she received another anti-emetic injection. Tomorrow, we assured her and ourselves, she must surely suffer a less violent reaction to the chemotherapy. Tomorrow *must* be easier.

The curtains had been pulled round Jane's bed to shut the world out as much as possible. The promised injection seemed to relieve her, and she slept at last.

The next day the sickness was slightly less, but Jane was having difficulty with her tongue, which lolled out of her mouth. She couldn't swallow properly and mopped at her saliva. The doctor didn't seem concerned.

When Rosemary arrived early the following day – she had special permission to come before visiting hours – Jane was a frightening sight. Her tongue appeared even more swollen and sticking out of her mouth. She could only mumble. She managed to convey that she must drink; if she didn't, she'd have to be given another saline drip. The saliva dribbled uncontrollably from her mouth. She kept trying to drink the blackcurrant juice that Rosemary held to her lips, but she couldn't swallow. The paper tissues with which she feverishly mopped her mouth were stained purple; so were her lips and nightdress. Her eyes rolled in fear as she fought to swallow small mouthfuls of juice, failing again and again. She would signal for yet another tissue and frantically try to catch the liquid as it ran down the sides of her mouth, round her tongue and on to her neck.

Appalled, Rosemary asked for the doctor. He came quickly, but still appeared unconcerned, reiterating that Jane's tongue wasn't swollen. They would take an X-ray to find out what was wrong. It was hard to believe his detachment wasn't put on – perhaps to hide an inability to cope. Rosemary felt very frightened. Jane had motioned to her to draw the curtains round the bed. She did so. This was in fact a mistake. If the nurses and other patients in the ward had seen her continual distress, she would have been given help and support.

Rosemary thought of Victor flying from America that day and soon due to arrive at the hospital. She imagined his feelings at seeing Jane in such distress and decided to tell him not to come. Surely tomorrow she would be better. If this was what chemotherapy did for Jane, Rosemary swore to herself, there would be no more doses.

When she spoke to Victor on the phone, he insisted on coming straight to the hospital. His first sight of Jane in six months was a terrible moment for him. He put an arm round her in anguish. She tried to say something, but no words came out, only an incoherent mumble. As she returned his embrace, he was overcome with despair. What had they done to her? Then she spoke just one word, 'Dad . . .' He said, 'Jane,' and broke down. His face touched hers, and he could feel her tears on his cheek, as they mingled with his own.

The reunion was too painful for both of them. It made Rosemary realise how weak Jane had become. After a short time, Jane indicated that he should go. By now she was unable to produce even a whisper, only a breath of sound, and she pointed with her finger to make sure she was understood. But she wanted Rosemary to stay.

A porter arrived to take Jane down to the X-ray room in a wheelchair. Jane managed a feeble 'Nonsense!' but allowed herself to be helped into the chair and they set off, with her head lolling uncontrollably, her tongue protruding, the saliva dribbling.

The wait outside the X-ray room seemed endless. Finally the radiographers began their work – or attempted to. Jane had by now completely lost control of her head and shoulders which sagged helplessly. They tried to position her neck for an X-ray, but she couldn't hold her body in place as they took the picture. They tried again and again.

Then an emergency case required their attention and we were shifted to a tiny room like a cupboard, where we would be sheltered from the X-rays, to wait until the radiographers were free again. The door was closed. There was hardly space for the wheelchair. A single bulb hung from the ceiling, giving a dim light that added to the sense of anxiety in the small cell.

Rosemary struggled hard against the panic that threatened to overwhelm her. It was as if they were in limbo. Jane seemed to be slipping further and further away. She couldn't speak, but she intimated she felt sick. Rosemary pounded on the tightly closed door. Miraculously it opened, and a basin was handed in. They began to wonder if they would be there for ever.

When one of the radiographers opened the door again, Rosemary's nerve failed. She ran. The sight of her daughter degenerating into a total wreck, a sort of classic village idiot, head lolling, mouth drooling, with no help or comfort, was unbearable. She rushed back along the corridors, up the stairs, along more passages, running from terror, running for help.

She didn't stop until she saw the rest of the family standing at the entrance to the ward. Richard quickly grasped the situation and hurried with Joan to the X-ray room. Desperately, Rosemary turned to Victor.

'Calm down,' he said quietly. 'Things will get very much worse.'

She knew that this surface matter-of-factness was designed to hide his inner despair. She said nothing of her need for comfort because it seemed to her that there was none. He had spoken the truth.

Richard whisked Jane out of the X-ray room almost before the radiographers grasped what he was doing. Soon she was back in bed, surrounded by a team of nurses and doctors. They told us Jane must rest, we should go now. We returned to the flat, but all felt guilty that we had left Jane alone. Richard couldn't keep still, and finally asked Joan to go back to the hospital with him. They set off at once to find out what was happening.

The phone rang. Rosemary braced herself for more bad news, but it was Jane's voice, ringing clearly, full of happiness: 'Mum, I'm all right! They gave me an injection and it happened right away – I got human again!'

One of the doctors had recognised a very rare reaction to the anti-emetic drug. Neutralising it had been a simple matter. The chemotherapy could continue.

The evening before Richard and Joan left for Boston, friends had planned a party. Jane said that the family should leave the hospital early, before visiting hours were over. She would be fine, she insisted. Richard stayed with her for a few minutes longer. She kept up a brave front as she said good-bye. He couldn't tell her what was really on his mind. Instead he said: 'If you don't get to Boston to stay with us soon, I'll come over at the end of the summer.' Then he joined the rest of us and Jane was alone in the crowded ward.

As soon as he had gone, she broke down and wept for a long time.

That night she wrote in her diary: 'The reality of the possibility of my death has struck home to me in that I might not see Richard again – and although we've hardly seen much of each other in the last ten years I do feel very close to him and love him very much.'

Chapter 4

April was a time of public triumph in England: the country was getting ready to celebrate twenty-five years of the Queen's reign, her Jubilee. Flags flew everywhere, the monarch's smiling face looked out from photographs in shop windows and bookstalls. Posters hung across buildings carrying the triumphant message: 'Twenty-five Years.' The contrast between all the rejoicing and the realities of the twenty-fifth year of Jane's life was a terrible one. The decorations appeared tawdry to us, the sounds of festivity and triumph a mockery. The thousands of souvenirs that filled the shops seemed, for the most part, unforgivably ugly.

Jane saw little of all this. Two days after Richard and Joan went back to America, she was discharged from the hospital and came to the flat we had rented nearby, to be close to her after the operation. Not only was her body damaged by the disease but her confidence and sense of independence were gone. 'I just can't imagine myself driving again,' she said. 'All these cars, all these people . . . For that matter, I can't even see myself sitting in a bus!'

She had been continuously ill for nine weeks. Time dragged. TV bored her, even music began to pall. 'What can one do to make the time pass quickly?' she asked gloomily.

'Why not try that embroidery I bought for you?' said Rosemary, who was knitting furiously.

'It's too complicated. I looked at it, but it's too difficult.'

Rosemary went shopping and chose a pattern of sunflowers for needlepoint. The design was pleasing, the colours all went together. Jane began to work at once. She would sit for hours pushing the needle through the canvas, in and out. Building up the design of flowers and leaves was relaxing and finishing a flower or a corner of the pattern rewarding. At last she had something to show that she'd done herself.

Slowly Jane began to eat properly; slowly her strength returned. She started to cook, to talk of going out one day. Soon she was able to negotiate the flights of stairs down from the flat and cross the road to the little park – but not for long, and not alone. She still needed support, both physical and psychological.

A visit to the café near the hospital after treatment was a big event. A trip out to dinner with Michael, who took her to an Indian restaurant that had many associations for them, was a real milestone.

But getting Jane interested in the future was still hard going. She felt the best she had to look forward to was a short life full of chemotherapy – a year of treatment, perhaps several years if no more tumours appeared. She wanted to earn a living by teaching; she didn't want to exist on her parents' charity. But who would employ her as a teacher, with one week off every month for chemotherapy, and goodness knows how much more time for the various other disabilities that might lurk in the unknown? 'Who would want someone with cancer?' she asked.

'The way to look at it,' Victor told her, 'is not to decide whether *they* want you, but what you want to work at, then go ahead and get on with it.'

'You know very well I'm in no position to act like that,' she replied angrily.

'But ignore that for a moment, Jane,' Victor persisted. 'Let's look at it as if it were an intellectual exercise. There must be other work than teaching that would interest you.'

She was still angry, but said nothing. This was like one of their exchanges when she was a teenager.

'All right, granted it's difficult for you to imagine now that you could be holding down a real job. Let's talk about some of the things you'd like to have done in the past, not jobs so much as things you'd enjoy – travelling, perhaps, or writing?'

'You always said I shouldn't go into journalism. You're

not going to change your mind now, just to humour me?'
Her tone was sarcastic.

'No, but you could write. There's your poetry. There's women's rights. Your dissertation on that was pretty good.'

'No, Dad, I want something I could *live* on.'

'But before you discover that, you've got to find something you can do – that you want to do and can do. Something worth doing, fulfilling. Didn't you once want to bring art to the people?'

'What on earth are you talking about?' She was less angry now than impatient, and a little curious.

'I remember a conversation you and Mum once had in the pottery. You were putting her pots on the shelves, preparing for a sale. You told her you knew how she liked it when local people bought her pots, not just her rich friends.'

'Well, so what?'

'And you agreed with her that what Granny used to call "the lower classes" were quite as capable of appreciating the finer crafts as anyone, when they got a chance to see good work. Do you remember that?'

'Yes,' she acknowledged grudgingly. 'But what's all that got to do with us now?'

'Just this – you said that maybe you and Mum should go into partnership, that she could make pots and you should sell them – pottery, woodwork, things like that, at the right prices, to the right people, and bring something into their lives that they'd appreciate, instead of the plastic rubbish people often buy because shops don't stock anything better.'

'But it would cost a lot of money, a shop like that.' Jane eyed him dubiously. 'And I'd still have to shut it for a week every month, during chemotherapy, and at any other time I didn't feel well. No, Dad, thanks, but it isn't very practical.'
Now she was no longer angry, only a little sad.

But Victor was relentless. 'You could borrow the money, and repay it out of your earnings. You'd be able to hire an assistant or take a partner to be in charge in your absence. If we found you a place in Brighton, all your friends there would rally round. You could have a flat over the shop, so that you'd know what was going on even if you couldn't always be there. And Mum has been talking about staying on in England with you for a while – she could have a pottery in the back.'

It was then that Jane called out to Rosemary, 'Mum! Mum!' Her voice ran with a vitality we had not heard for many weeks. Rosemary came quickly in from the kitchen: 'Yes, Jane, what is it?'

'Dad's had one of his ideas.'

'Well, what is it this time?' Rosemary asked warily. Victor's 'ideas' were usually big and rarely practical.

But Jane's excitement as she described the Brighton idea was infectious. Brighton was the place where she had been happy, during her university days, and she had often gone back there to see the friends who had stayed on. Could she recapture those times again? Soon the three of us were sitting at the table with pencils and paper making lists: Victor of people to phone; Rosemary of potters and other craftsmen to see; Jane of things to do, from the renting of premises to the buying of stock, from finding out about taxation to making visits to other shops to see how they were run. We planned it almost like a military campaign. Jane supplied the sense of order, the realism; she asked the difficult questions, and insisted on a proper sequence of actions. Victor added the enthusiasm, excitement, ideas. In no time at all he was talking, only half-jokingly, of a chain of shops scattered through the slum areas of Britain, bringing arts and crafts to the people there. Jane smiled indulgently. 'First, catch your hare, Dad' – Mrs. Beaton's cookbook injunction had become a family saying long ago. Rosemary gave practical advice, happy because Jane seemed happy, which was all that mattered.

Was it only a charade? Jane's chances that day were no better than they had been twenty-four hours before. She had again wakened with a pain in her back, and we knew that persistent pain could signify the return of the cancer. We knew it, but it was not something we could bring ourselves to talk about.

In her diary, Jane wrote: 'I'm getting better, but it is a frustrating, slow business. I feel I have so much to cope with – now, in the next year, and for the rest of my life. First of all, I have to accept that the cancer may return, and that my chances of dying are considerably higher than is normal for someone of my age – and that it appears that no one can or will tell me just what the chances of it recurring are. Then, I have to accept the fact of my physical weakness: it has never been as bad before, but at least I have started to eat, and I'm able to move around more, though it's still very little. Then, there is the chemotherapy – it shouldn't be as bad again as it was the first time, but it's not going to be pleasant. It will take up a week every month for about a year, and it'll make me pretty ill. And there are the problems that will have to be faced when I have recovered more from my operations and the treatments: how can I possibly find a job, with the continuing need for treatment? Is it viable for me to live indefinitely at Dairy Cottage with my parents?

'And there is the knowledge that for a long time I'm going to be on the receiving end, and getting emotional and practical support from family and friends.'

The day after the 'Brighton project' was born, her diary entry was much more cheerful: 'Despite my cold, I am really beginning to feel well again. I can finally walk across a room without feeling faint. As I get physically better, it becomes easier to feel optimistic. Last night was the first time I slept without waking up with a severe stomach ache. My diarrhoea seems to be over, too. . . . A major factor in my improvement, which is both physical and mental, is a new Zorza plan. Dad says he is happy and willing to provide money for me to set up a craft shop which will probably be in the Brighton area. Of course, it would not be an easy project, and there is an awful lot to find out about, and a lot of work involved – but it really seems as if it might work out.'

Together, she and Rosemary set out to visit a number of craft shops. Jane carried a notebook from one display case to another, writing down the names of craftsmen who caught her fancy, comments on their work, comparisons of prices. She was deciding what proportion of her stock would consist of pottery, woodwork, glassware.

Jane put together a list of good craftsmen in the Brighton area, and some further afield, whose work she might want to stock, but not before she had carefully studied slides, pictures, and some actual examples of their products. They didn't all pass muster. 'That may be good enough for one of the big London shops, but not for mine.' Her energy was amazing.

She got into long discussions about standards, quality, and price. 'I want to stock things that are both functional and beautiful,' she wrote to Teresa, 'and a few that are simply beautiful. But there is a problem, in that I want things ordinary people can afford – and a lot of craft-work, especially in textiles, is very expensive.' This was where Carol, from the Crafts Advisory Council's London headquarters, could be very helpful. Carol was a new friend she made while trying to get the shop organised. Many of the young, struggling potters whom Carol was trying to support were quite as good as some of the better known ones and their prices were often much lower. Jane saw herself befriending some of these young people, providing an outlet for them, perhaps guiding them in reconciling their artistic drive with the dictates of the market. This would be a market she would create, and it would be governed not by the philistine views of the undiscerning, but by the down-to-earth, practical appreciation of the functional and the beautiful which, she insisted, would be the mark of her own customers.

She knew all this would take time, a long time, and she talked of how the various stages of the project would have to mature gradually, of the transitions from one stage to the next, of the slow growth of her relationship with the craftsmen who would be her suppliers first, and then perhaps her friends. But how long? That she didn't go into – and neither did we. Did she really believe it was possible? We never knew.

She wrote to Teresa: 'The sun is shining, the birds are singing, and the world is very, very beautiful. . . . I'm in my usual state of exhaustion, but we've had a good afternoon looking at the British Craft Centre shop, and a place called the Glasshouse, where people make and sell glass.' The visit to the Glasshouse, with its great glowing furnace and its glassmakers blowing into their long pipes, had excited her. It was one of her most enjoyable experiences in a long time.

'We saw some beautiful glassware – but quite expensive. And we watched a goblet being made – fascinating, despite the fact that I was suffering, as I have been for days, with painful shoulders.' Not even those few golden days were free of painful reminders. She tried not to let them interfere with her Brighton dream, but occasoinly she began to doubt that there was enough time left. And then she would ask bitterly how she could run the shop if she were going to be in pain all the time.

She wrote to Teresa: 'Of course, the shop project hasn't managed to make me forget all about the cancer. I think that would be unhealthy. I just have to live with the possibility of a recurrence and make the best of things. It gets easier, with time, and is easier now that I have something I really want to do. I do feel so much more optimistic about things.'

On her bad days, she didn't give up the idea but raised all kinds of doubts. What if she got a loan from a bank and borrowed money from Victor, and then had to go back into hospital? What if she simply couldn't go through with it, after spending a lot of money setting up the shop? She didn't say, 'What if I die soon?' but that was clearly on her mind.

Victor felt he had to meet this objection to keep up her interest in the shop – and maintain the feeling that she had a future.

'You can't measure in money the satisfaction this project will bring you,' he insisted. 'It's already brought you happiness while we've been working on it just these past couple of weeks, and that's what matters. It's worth all the money it's going to cost to have made you as happy as you have been since we began this. Anything more will be just a bonus. . . .'

That was as close as he could bring himself to discuss the possibility of her dying. She seemed to accept what he said and to be ready to go on. Negotiations for a building and a bank loan began. But her doubts revived as the pain returned.

'Are you sure you want to go through with it, Dad?' she asked. 'Is it really worth it? You don't have to, you know.' Did she think Victor was reluctant to spend the money; that the new pain made him feel it would be wasted, that she was going to die? There had been times in her childhood when we needed to be very careful about money. He did his best to convince her, feeling guilty about the past.

But Jane's bouts of depression didn't last long, and they were greatly outweighed by bursts of sustained enthusiasm. 'My own feelings,' she wrote in her diary, 'vary between great enthusiasm, a belief that it really will work, and doubts as to whether I am able to undertake the considerable work and responsibility.' But, she added, 'it's almost worrying, how well things have gone.'

When Richard had left at the beginning of April she was concerned that she might never see him again. By the end of the month, she could write to him: 'I wish you could see me now. It's unbelievable, how much better I am. . . . We think we might be able to open in July or August, but a lot depends on how much the treatment knocks me out, on how soon we get premises, on how long it will take to get stock, etc. But the whole process is so enjoyable – I now lie awake at night thinking of the shop and all that, rather than about the cancer.'

For a short time she seemed to be full of hope. Even Richard ceased insisting that she should be told how remote were her chances of survival. We were affected by her enthusiasm, and wondered if some real recovery could be possible. Our guilt was eased. If she had been told she was under sentence of death, her present happiness would have been impossible. But we were also worried that perhaps it was a false happiness, based on lies and concealment, and that she might have used her time to better purpose.

We could never be sure what to do. All we knew was that Jane did seem happy. She didn't actually tell us so, because in the midst of resolving the practical problems raised by the Brighton project there was no talk about feelings, hers or ours. It might have been a dangerous topic. We didn't want to risk spoiling things.

But she confessed in her diary explicitly what we only guessed at.

'It has given me something to live for.' She was 'a real person again – hopefully, even more real' than before her illness. More real, because her heightened sensitivity made it possible to perceive her own feelings and those of others in a way she had never done before. She had a unique vantage point that allowed her to explore the depth and richness of human values and relationships, of the world's beauty. 'I feel I have learned quite a lot that maybe I knew intellectually before, but not emotionally. In a way it's made me more selfish, more determined to live the way I want to live *now* and not think too much of doing things in the future. And I appreciate things (the beautiful ones, anyway) and people (the nice ones) much more.'

This enhanced appreciation of beauty, which was evident in her search for objects for the shop, and in her delight – a mixture of the sophisticated and the childlike – when she found them, was something she could share with others, not just her parents. When she handled a piece of wood that had been lovingly fashioned by a craftsman, when she looked at a picture of a pot from a prospective supplier, there was an almost sensual pleasure in her response which communicated itself to those around her. Sometimes a shop manager who had seemed busy and harried would be drawn into her little circle of light, take time to admire with her an object on his shelf, discuss its finer points –and, on discovering she was a prospective shopkeeper, offer sage advice and practical warnings.

In Brighton the first bank manager she had ever dealt with extensively was willing to give as much time as she wanted to discuss comparatively minor points with her. He was aware she had cancer, which to him meant she was not long for this world, and he felt she knew it. He was shaken by her calm and marvelled at her practical approach, but was careful to hide his feelings. Yet she knew what he was doing. 'I'm learning new things all the time,' she said. 'Bank managers *are* human. No, not just human, that's a cliché, they're like you and me. They *feel*.'

There was the man who had recently closed down his own crafts shop in Brighton and was prepared to sell Jane very cheaply the remainder of his stock, the goodwill of his business, and the detailed information about his suppliers and customers it might have taken her years to acquire. It wasn't a business deal to him – or to her. His heart went out to Jane, to a fellow human being facing the pain of cancer and the mystery of existence, and he offered help and friendship at a time when she needed it. What he was giving her was hope that her project was realistic, that it would work.

Jane's new friends were all nice to her, even the young man who argued heatedly with her, maintaining – as she might have done a few years before – that it was a petit bourgeois illusion to believe that working people needed access to art and the crafts. He ridiculed her idea of 'going to the people' with the precious gift of beauty, when what they really needed was power – power to remake society, power to take away from the rich their monopoly on power itself. Only then could the people gain a true appreciation of beauty.

She explained to him, using his own vocabulary, why she thought that working people already had an appreciation of beauty, and why she could see it as a worthwhile life's work to help them develop and deepen that appreciation. She would make it possible for them to have beautiful things. Their lives would be the richer for it, and so would her own.

'Yes,' he retorted. 'Of course it will. You'll grow rich on it all right. Money-grabbing, that's what it is. You'll be a shop-keeper – you, with your fine ideals!'

She was not in the least put out by the encounter. She went from one Brighton estate agent to another, looking at the premises she had arranged to view when she telephoned them from London to explain exactly what she wanted. She was searching for something in one of the poorer shopping areas, where the kind of customer she was after was likely to be passing by. Finally, after nearly two days of dragging herself through the streets of Brighton, the pain in her shoulders getting worse and worse, having to sit down more and more often, but without a single complaint, she found it. The space was in a street that also contained a market, so she would have the clientele she wanted; but she would have more than that.

'Do you see that shop at the other end of the street, on the corner?' she asked us. That, she explained, was Infinity, a health food co-op that was now the best shop of its kind in town, attracting a lot of the middle-class customers of exactly the kind, she said shrewdly, that her place might deal with while she was building up her own special clientele.

'That could take a long time,' she said, looking Victor

straight in the eye. 'I may not be able to make it, but it's worth trying. If I can get that shop, Dad, it will have been worth having had cancer.'

She waited for him to reply, but he couldn't bring himself to say anything. It was the first time she had acknowledged how fragile the project might turn out to be.

'Infinity – that's a good name,' she went on. 'I wish the co-op hadn't grabbed it. It would have suited us fine, don't you think?'

Still he could say nothing.

'But perhaps we can improve on it,' she continued. 'Something even more suitable . . . I think I've got it. We'll call it "Close to Infinity". What do you think?' she asked with a smile.

'Yes, Jane, that sounds fine,' he said flatly.

'Oh, come on, Dad. It sounds better than fine. It sums it all up, doesn't it? That's where I am, and that's where I'll remain, from now on. *Close to Infinity.*'

Jane grew steadily stronger, more confident. One day she arranged to travel across London to visit Michael. She was determined to make the journey on her own, but asked Rosemary to accompany her to the doors of the Underground while she got her courage up to continue alone. Then she said : 'If you could just buy me a paper, then I can read it all the way and not get claustrophobic in the train.' Armed with the paper, she waved goodbye like a child determined to act the adult, and disappeared into the subway.

When Michael opened the door of his house some time later, he was delighted to find her on the doorstep. The old Jane had come back to him – alone, tired, but on her feet and radiantly happy to have reached him unaided. It was a moment of natural celebration. He welcomed her with a delight that equalled her own. He put his arms round her, drawing her into an embrace that she returned happily. He led her into the house, and it was as if nothing had ever come between them. They picked up the threads of their student days in Brighton, reliving the old pleasures, renewing the intimacy of a past life.

Michael shared the house with friends, some of whom had also been part of their lives in Brighton. But Jane's illness wasn't mentioned, it was treated as part of the past and ignored. Michael had always fought for Jane's individuality, anxious she shouldn't become an object, a cancer sufferer with no identity other than 'sick'. Now the battle seemed won. She was 'Jane' again, full of life, both living in the present and looking forward to the future. They cooked and ate with their friends, reliving the old rituals of a shared life, listening to much-loved records of the Grateful Dead on the same old stereo, smoking. Alone together in the happiness of that night they made love.

The threat she was living under, although suppressed in their conscious thoughts, was never very far from the surface of their minds. But that night, 'we made it go away,' Michael recalled later. There was a sense of rejoicing about the occasion as they rolled back the months of illness and of separation to seize the time to be lovers again. It did not come easily, at first, and they were both a little shy. They talked a good deal, slowly feeling their way back to the simple physical intimacy they had once known. Jane gradually regained confidence about her disease-ravaged body. Michael had thought about her operations, about the scars she would still be bearing, about the pain she might feel, but he had also determined to show his love for her however her body might be altered. 'I didn't in my head want to make love because of my wound,' Jane wrote in her diary later, 'but my body wanted to.' Michael sensed her uncertainty and her need to be shown that she was a full person, for he knew how grievously someone in her condition might suffer in the absence of such reassurance. It proved easier than he had expected. 'Look what they've done to me,' she said, as she showed him her scars. It wasn't important. He wanted to express his feelings towards her; he was determined that she should understand what they were – and he knew that this could be achieved best by making love. 'If you love somebody enough,' he was to say later, 'you can forget other things. The very words you use, the way you can be together – all this takes you out of yourself, it transcends the present. That's how it was with me and Jane.'

It was the best night's sleep Jane had enjoyed in a long while, and without sleeping pills – a great achievement. She woke with a smile and stayed in bed late, happy and relaxed. They talked of her plans, of the Brighton project, but as if by agreement their conversation touched only on the present and the immediate future. Michael, for all his refusal to face the facts, felt subconsciously that this might be their last time together, even though this was at odds with the conscious and deliberate effort he was making to help her act and behave as a normal, healthy human being. There was, for him, the joy of something new opening up – and, at the same time, the sense that a door might be closing forever.

For Jane, there was the triumph of her body's victory over its ills. With a new confidence, she refused Michael's offer to call a cab for her, and insisted that she would walk unaccompanied to the Underground.

When she got home from seeing Michael and the pain reminded her of her uncertain future, Jane too could see the door opening – and shutting. 'I now feel that I do want some sort of a relationship with him,' she wrote in her diary, 'but will be unable to have it.' She felt very close to him. 'If any one person can supply a lot of my needs – for a good friend to talk to, for a lover, or companion – for some of the time, not all of it – then it is him. But I feel I don't have much to give him in return, and that's no basis for a relationship.' She was depressed again, experiencing one of those periods of dejection when the future seemed bleak, if indeed, there was to be a future.

But the pain in her shoulders began to grow. At first it was referred to as Jane's 'backache' or 'rheumatism'. When it was worse, perhaps weather was to blame. If it rained in the morning, Victor would remark that Jane's rheumatism would be bad. When she complained, we wondered aloud if she shouldn't see a specialist, but we didn't press the matter. None of us really wanted her to see a doctor. Once it was discovered she didn't have rheumatism, the straw Jane was clutching would be gone and we could no longer help her deceive herself.

It was a relief when night came. Sleeping pills often helped, if only for a few hours. She usually awoke early, but one morning she still hadn't made a sound by ten o'clock. The sleep would do her good – she obviously needed it. Whenever we went past her room, we tiptoed. Victor rushed out to meet the postman in case he rang the doorbell. Rosemary shut the kitchen door when she did the dishes. So long as Jane was asleep, she wasn't in pain. We were also freed a little longer from playing our game of deception. The pain was making her irritable – that and perhaps the realisation that Brighton was just a dream. She was getting on our nerves, and she knew it. Several times she had told us what a burden she was. She said it almost angrily, not apologetically as she might have done in the past. Her incessant cigarette smoking left a smell of stale tobacco in the house and we struggled to accept it. Smoking was a great relief for her, and it was little enough to put up with compared to her pain, but so long as she was asleep, we were free of this too.

As noon approached, Jane still hadn't woken up. Victor no longer bothered to walk on tiptoe. He put on a Mozart record, one of her favourites, hoping it would make her awakening more pleasant. Still there was no sound from upstairs.

Suddenly the telephone rang. Jane was a light sleeper, that would surely waken her. Victor let the phone ring until it stopped, but she didn't respond.

Rosemary stood outside her door and listened. 'Not a sound,' she confirmed; she was no longer whispering. 'If Jane is still asleep, then that means she needs to sleep.'

Victor looked thoughtful. 'Supposing she took more sleeping pills than usual, should we just leave her?'

Rosemary didn't answer at once. She led him away from Jane's door into the sitting room. 'Let's give her a little more time,' she said gently. Victor let himself be guided to the sofa, feeling suddenly powerless. 'She has slept as late as this?'

'No, never,' Rosemary said nervously. 'But then, she's not been in quite this kind of state before, has she?' She was remembering her conversation about suicide with Jane, but all she said to Victor was, 'Let's leave her alone. Let her sleep.'

'Yes,' Victor agreed. 'She must have taken more pills than usual to sleep as deeply as this.'

'There's certainly enough in that bottle to knock her out, if that's what she wanted.'

He took a deep breath. 'Knock her right out?'

'If she wanted to, yes.'

He wasn't ready to face it. He backtracked a little. 'Then she wouldn't want us to wake her now. She'd bite our heads off, as she did when you offered her breakfast yesterday.'

'She seemed much happier last night. When I helped her to bed, she said: "Let's go shopping – I know I've had such a lot of presents, but it's been so long since I *chose* something."'

Victor felt more confused. That didn't sound like someone about to take an overdose. But Rosemary was pursuing her own train of thought. 'Perhaps when the pain became worse, as it always does at night, when she couldn't sleep for hours, she'd have got more depressed than before.'

'You think that would be enough to make her take an extra dose of sleeping pills?'

'Perhaps she woke in the night . . .'

He put his arm around her. 'Yes,' he said. 'She'd think another night of pain, and another, and another . . .'

Rosemary took his hand, ready to answer his question now. 'It would be enough to make her take an extra dose,' she said quietly, 'or an overdose.'

There – it was out.

Victor stroked her hand.

'Or an overdose,' he repeated, then paused. 'That's what I've been thinking for some time now.'

'Yes, I know. So have I.'

'It'd be for the best this way,' Rosemary said. Victor drew her towards him and kissed her. 'Yes,' he said. 'She has a right to do what she wants.'

'It's her life.'

'If we tried to stop her, we'd be doing it for our sakes, not hers.'

We'd made our decision, but we needed to reassure one another, to give each other the strength to go through with it.

'She won't feel anything by now,' Rosemary said.

'No, but we must give her as long as possible.'

'Yes. We must make sure.'

We sat . . . waiting.

It was twelve o'clock, then one. Then a new thought hit Rosemary – hard. What if Jane had tried and failed? What if she was lying upstairs half-conscious, unable to move or call out, desperate for help?

For the first time that morning communication between us broke down. Rosemary threw Victor a wild glance and rushed upstairs. He started to follow her, but couldn't face what lay in the bedroom. A memory came into his mind of Jane as a happy child, playing with other children, her face smudged with dirt, lit up with a puckish smile.

He heard the bedroom door open and Rosemary go in. There was a brief silence, then he heard Jane's 'Oh,' as she woke up. She came to slowly and reluctantly, and seemed very cross at being woken. She was in pain and said little for the rest of the day, remaining withdrawn, almost hostile. When Rosemary brought her some food, she pushed it angrily away.

'If this goes on,' she snapped, 'I shall have to do myself in.'

Rosemary could say nothing.

Chapter 5

'How's the pain?' Rosemary asked.

'Foul.'

'Did the hot water bottle help last night?'

'It made it worse.'

The day before, Victor had massaged Jane, rubbing ointment into her shoulders, and she said it helped her rheumatism. But now nothing was any use. When Victor touched her back, she screamed: 'Don't touch me! Let's go to the hospital. There must be something they can do about rheumatism.'

An appointment was made for the next afternoon, but the pain was suddenly so intense that Jane felt she couldn't wait that long.

'No, not tomorrow. Now! *Now!*'

When Victor finally got through to the hospital again, the doctor Jane was to see the next day was away.

'But Jane can't wait,' he spluttered. 'She's got to see someone. Today.'

'It's too late. She'll have to come in tomorrow for her appointment.'

'No, no, *please*.' Victor knew he couldn't go back to Jane with this news. He said desperately, 'She's talking of doing away with herself.'

There was a brief silence at the other end. Then: 'Bring her in now, but straight away. Hurry, before the clinic ends. Can you make it in an hour?'

They just made it, but then they had to wait another hour before the nurse called Jane's name. She had hardly spoken during the drive, except to grunt with exasperation when

Victor braked sharply and made her wince with pain. She didn't say anything in the waiting room.

She was soon back from the examination, bursting in, furious, on the point of crying not with pain, but with anger.

'You go and see him! You talk to him and tell him what they said!' she almost shouted at Victor, heedless of the other patients.

'What happened? Tell him what who said?'

'Go on! Go!'

A doctor was waiting inside. Distressed, he told Victor, 'She's very touchy. It's only to be expected. Something I said must obviously have upset her. Do you know what it was?'

'What *did* you say to her?'

'I told her there's nothing we could do about her pain. It's something she must expect in a case like this. She knows what she's got. If she can learn to accept it, it'll be easier for her.'

Victor looked at him, shocked. 'You told her *that*?'

'That's all I could say to her, based on her case history, on my own experience.'

'But they said it might be something else,' Victor protested. ' "Rheumatism," they said. "Give it a little time, it might go away." '

The doctor picked up the folder with Jane's name on it, examined the last page, then looked at Victor.

'There's nothing about rheumatism here.'

'Maybe it's in another file? We were definitely told that. No wonder she was upset.'

'I see.' The doctor paused. 'Well, she'd better see her own doctor, who'll be back in a day or two. I can only tell you what I know.'

When Victor returned to Jane, she still wouldn't talk to him. She heard what he had to say – that the doctor had based his remarks on the contents of her file, which seemed incomplete – but made no comment. Her anger had subsided; she appeared to have lost interest. When she got home, she pushed silently past Rosemary, who was anxious for news. Rosemary followed upstairs and helped her into bed. What had the doctor said?

'Oh, I lost patience with him. He didn't know anything about my case . . .'

The next day they were ready for her. She was whisked into a large consulting room, where two or three other patients were already being examined. A nurse who had been offhand the day before was now very attentive, almost tender, helping her to lie down. The doctors were equally caring. Jane submitted passively to their exhaustive examination. The anger of the day before seemed spent. For once, she hadn't prepared her usual list of questions, and none seemed to occur to her while she was being examined.

Victor asked about the rheumatism when Jane was out of earshot, but he was given no direct answer. 'We ought to get some specialists to see her,' said one of the doctors vaguely. 'More tests will be necessary to track down the cause of the pain.' It would be better if she came back into hospital. She'd been very upset at home, hadn't she? That kind of pain could be disturbing, unnerving, and could affect people in odd ways . . .

When Victor told Jane that the doctors wanted her back, it was obvious she knew already, that she had heard everything. Victor felt that the doctors should have been more judicious, but Jane didn't seem to care. A mask of indifference hid her feelings, even when one of the doctors said she should be admitted immediately.

She lay on the bench in the waiting room for well over an hour while the bed was being prepared, saying nothing, hardly stirring. When they finally came, she rose with a great effort, supported by Victor and a nurse. That morning she had needed no support. Now she was dependent on other people, ready to collapse without them. She had become an invalid again.

Her bed was in a nearby ward occupied mostly by old women. They eyed Jane curiously as she tried to get undressed. But soon a nurse pulled the curtain round the bed and helped her into it. When the curtain was pulled back, Jane was lying down, seemingly lifeless, her eyes shut.

That day we realised she was withdrawing from us. When we tried to talk, she would not respond. When we asked questions, she would not answer. For the first time since her illness began, she was concerned that we should keep to the visiting hours. We should leave, she told us. It was past the time for visitors; it wasn't fair to the other patients.

We left reluctantly, without any warm goodbye from Jane. Looking back, we traced the beginning of this new mood to that morning she had slept late. From then on, she seemed to have become sullen, almost hostile towards us. She protected herself with a wall of silence. More sensitive to her daughter's signals than Victor, Rosemary saw such behaviour as a need on Jane's part to assert herself, to show that she hadn't relapsed into total dependence again. Victor could accept this intellectually, but he was nevertheless very hurt by the withdrawal.

Next morning he returned to the hospital, expecting Jane to have recovered from her gloom. But when he greeted her cheerfully, she barely responded. It was the same the following day. She made it quite clear by her behaviour during the ensuing days that she didn't want us there. We took turns in sitting with her, but she hardly acknowledged our presence. When we offered her something – a drink, fruit, a magazine – she would curtly reject it. But when the nurse came by, she would often ask for the very thing she had just refused from us. We developed a guilt complex. What had we done wrong? It was obvious to us that, in spite of Jane's rejection, she needed us as much as she had in the other crises of her life, even more so. There had been times in the past when she was angry with us, but we'd stuck it out, and after the storm blew over were glad we had done so. We would stick it out this time, too.

We were back in the days of Jane's adolescence, when her moods, the alternating periods of depression and rebellion, made her relapse into silence for days. 'Jane is off,' the family used to say, and leave her alone until she gave some sign of being 'on' again.

Now Rosemary looked for similar signals that Jane's depression was lifting, but all she saw were the old, familiar 'off' signs – the eyes-turned-to-heaven, the what-fools-I-have-for-parents expression. Real communication was difficult in any event because we didn't feel able to discuss Jane's chances realistically with her. We wanted to appear hopeful and encouraging, and this probably further irritated Jane when she was struggling to face the truth. She no longer mentioned rheumatism.

She was receiving no treatment at this time. Her second dose of chemotherapy had proved to be almost as bad as the first. The third course was not due for more than a week. Her rare remarks about these treatments made it possible to glimpse her deepest feelings. Rosemary, trying to get her to talk about the future, said: 'If you do get another tumour, then you won't have to go through chemotherapy again.' Jane replied flatly: 'I'd rather go on with chemotherapy and not have cancer, thank you.' Apparently she assumed that if another tumour appeared, further operations would be useless and only radiation and chemotherapy might help her. She knew the difference between the two – radiation would be directed at a particular tumour to shrink it and thus lessen the pain. But if the pain still continued, she seemed to conclude, this would prove that the treatment had failed, and then she would have no hope.

Not all Jane's assumptions were correct. Continued pain, for instance, would not necessarily mean that these two treatments had failed, for neither could succeed overnight. But to discuss this with her was difficult without raising the spectre of death – and that was a subject we carefully avoided at that time, though there were signs it was much on her mind.

Jane sometimes had to fight off nightmares by staying awake; but often the thoughts that came to her while she was awake were worse than the dreams. Was that why she had retired behind her wall of silence?

At home, when nightmares and pain tortured her in the night, one of us would get up to talk with her. But in the hospital there was no one to stay with her during the night. She was allowed to spend a weekend at home, yet now, in her withdrawn state, she came out of the hospital reluctantly, retired upstairs, and had little to say to us. But friends delighted her, and sounds of talking and laughter would come through the closed door. Then, when the visitors left, silence would once more take over.

One night at home, seeing her light was on, Victor brought her a fresh lemon drink, and gradually they started talking.

Rosemary heard their voices and joined them. A conversation with Jane was too rare to be missed these days. Jane talked of the pain, of how they weren't able to do anything for her at the hospital, of how unhappy she was.

This gave Victor the opening he wanted. 'I know how worrying all this must be to you now, Jane, until they can establish precisely what is causing the pain.'

'Yes, I wish they could do something about it,' she answered, as if to say that she, too, didn't think it was due to cancer.

If he had experienced as much pain as she had, over as long a period, Victor said, he didn't know how he could have put up with it. He spoke of her endurance, her courage. She listened impassively. He recalled her second operation, which took place when he was in Washington, and told her how much he regretted not being with her then.

'Mum told me how you talked then about the possibility of dying and how you were prepared to accept it,' he went on. 'It helps sometimes to talk about things – shall we talk now?'

'No, there's nothing more to say,' she said sharply.

He tried again another way. 'We know how hard it is for you to speak to us these days. It's natural when things are so difficult. We thought we'd ask Richard to come over.'

'No, I don't want Richard now.'

'You know, Jane,' Rosemary put in, 'how good Richard is at finding things out from the doctors? Dad says he's got no skill at this game.'

'It isn't information I need. I just want them to *do* something. If Richard comes over now, I'll know I'm dying. That'll be why you've asked him to fly back. I don't want him here.'

She couldn't have spoken more plainly. She wasn't ready to die, she didn't want to talk about it, and she didn't want to be made to think that she might be dying. Her silences, her withdrawal from us, began to look like a defence against being told something she didn't want to hear. Our hospital visits were a constant reminder of what Victor had blurted out – that she was dying. By driving us away from her, she perhaps would avoid any confirmation of her deepest suspicions that this might be true.

So far the new tests had revealed nothing. The doctors refused to commit themselves. There was no evidence of a tumour, and some of them, when asked, did not rule out rheumatism as a possibility. If we wanted to deceive ourselves, they were willing to help. They urged us to distract her, to stop her brooding about cancer. Take her shopping, said one doctor. Get her a lovely new dress. Another suggested a trip to Paris. 'There's a young man in the next ward who did just that. He went on holiday to France to enjoy himself, to forget everything – and it worked.'

Their attitude came close to telling Jane that she was making a fuss over nothing, that her pain wasn't as bad as she claimed.

'You sit there with a long face all the time,' said one doctor to Victor. 'It doesn't do anyone any good.' There was a danger that Jane would see in our patience with her bitchiness merely pity – and confirmation that her time was up.

We knew something of her thoughts from what she told other visitors, but she was selective in what she said to them. She sensed that some thought she was dying, and to those she would acknowledge in a matter-of-fact way that she, too, knew the truth. But she would insist that she hadn't given up hope, that she was determined to fight on, that there was chemotherapy, radiation, and perhaps other treatments which might help.

To those who didn't want to know, she would talk casually about everyday things, about her surroundings, about what was happening in their own lives. With them she was amiable, pleasant, composed, almost lighthearted at times.

Sometimes these friends acted as go-betweens. To James, a writer and an old family friend who had done much to encourage Jane's early ambitions as a poet, she spoke not only of her own suffering but also of what it was doing to her parents. Tanya, who had been seriously ill herself and still suffered considerable pain, quickly established an understanding with Jane on the basis of shared experience. But Tanya was also a mother, with a grown-up daughter, and she was therefore able to convey to Jane something of our own feelings about her rejection of us. Jane's remarks to these friends were reported back to us, as she knew they would be. Sometimes her messages were conciliatory; sometimes they were angry and bitter. When neither of us came one day, she told James that we must both be 'worn out'. She knew she was putting us under too much strain, she said, and she was concerned about us.

'I do like to see them every day,' she said, 'but I sometimes behave so badly. There are times I feel angry and take it out on them. I'm aware I'm doing it.'

She blamed it on the drugs, which made her constipated and irritable. 'They're the only people I can treat naturally, and they'll still come back. If I'm ever going to get through this, it's not by being goody-goody and accepting it all. I must fight it, resist it . . . Being a bitch sometimes gives me the strength to fight. It's the same as when someone says "Fuck you". It's meaningless, really, but . . . Well, there's a line in Shakespeare somewhere I remember from school. It "screws your courage to the sticking place" to get angry sometimes. Fuck you, cancer!'

To another visitor she acknowledged none of this, and expressed mainly anger at her parents. If they had to visit her, they should do so and then go, not hang around the hospital endlessly. Yes, she did turn her head deliberately to the wall when they came, because she didn't want them there. She was infuriated when they wouldn't take the hint and leave. They were a drain on her strength. Then, as if aware this might be hurtful, she sought to soften her remarks. She wanted to see them, but she didn't want to take up all their time. They had their own lives to live.

What were we to make of these conflicting messages? Did she need Victor there as a whipping boy, as she seemed to imply to James, or was our presence as burdensome as she had made out to others? We knew that much of her attitude grew out of 'displacement anger', as it was called in the books about dying which we had been reading for crumbs of comfort and advice. But it was still hard to accept.

One afternoon Rosemary stood by Jane's bed, looking out of the window and wondering what on earth she could say to break the long silence. Jane was reading a book – or more likely pretending to. Suddenly she spoke without looking up.

'Mum, I think you'd better go, and stay away for a day or two.'

It was the first time she had said it in so many words. Rosemary answered in the same matter-of-fact flat voice, 'Do you want Dad to come?'

'No, you'd better both stay away.'

Rosemary felt as if something had snapped inside her. The rejection was out in the open. She kissed Jane's unresponsive cheek, and told her to get someone to phone if she changed her mind.

She walked fast, very fast, down the long corridor, down the endless staircases. She found a phone and called Victor.

He was aghast. 'You haven't left her, have you? You can't. You mustn't. She needs us. Remember that book we read? It says that love and support must continue in the face of rejection. The book says . . .'

'I don't care what the book says! If I'm told to go, I go. How can I possibly stay?'

She left the hospital and turned through the crowded streets to a nearby park. She walked about for an hour, crying silently until she felt able to go home.

A message from the hospital awaited her there. A friend who'd been visiting Jane reported that she'd like to see Rosemary and Victor the next day.

Yet when we arrived next morning, there was no smile, no apology. She was polite, that was all. Most of our attempts at conversation were rebuffed. She asked Victor icily why he looked so glum. When he tried to be cheerful, she told him to stop pretending.

'Do you want me to leave?' he asked, irritated.

'Yes, and you'd better stay away.'

He managed to restrain his anger, but on the way home he shot the traffic lights and almost collided with another car. So that was how she was repaying everything they had done for her. It was time they took a stand, made it clear they wouldn't put up with her rudeness. She didn't want to see them? All right, she wouldn't! That would teach her a quick, sharp lesson.

Eventually he cooled down. One of the books we were reading was *On Death and Dying* by Elizabeth Kübler-Ross, who summed up our own situation when she spoke of patients who received their families' visits with little cheerfulness and anticipation. This, she commented, could make the encounter a very painful event. The family would either respond with grief and tears, guilt or shame, or avoid future visits, which would only increase the patient's discomfort or anger.

We both understood and were prepared for this, but when it happened the knowledge didn't alleviate our distress.

Kübler-Ross had written: 'The tragedy is perhaps that we do not think of the reasons for the patient's anger and take it personally, when it has originally little or nothing to do with the people who become the target of the anger. As the staff or family react personally to this anger, however, they respond with increasing anger on their part, only feeding into the patient's hostile behaviour.' Victor had read this passage several times, yet he had still taken Jane's attitude personally. He felt angry not at Jane but at himself.

The book was useful, however. Kübler-Ross wrote of the grief, shame and guilt felt by the family of a dying patient. The process of grief always included some qualities of anger. 'And who, in anger, had not at times wished someone would disappear, go away, or even dared to say: "Drop dead"?'

It helped us to know that our feelings were not unique even if it didn't help us to contain our anger. It wasn't something we could easily discuss with others. The doctors were mainly concerned with the physical aspects of the disease, and even the most sympathetic, helpful ones rarely had time for the kind of relaxed conversation that would allow us to bring our feelings into the open. Nor was it easy to tell friends how angry we sometimes felt. The books which dealt with such problems were helpful to us, but could also be misleading. Too great a reliance on the printed word proved dangerous, although on balance we gained understanding, comfort and practical advice from such books.

At first we insisted on sitting with Jane and sharing her silences, thinking we were doing what was best for her. When the silences turned into an angry rejection, we went back to Kübler-Ross. She wrote of patients who were depressed and morbidly uncommunicative until spoken to frankly about the terminal stage of their illness. 'Their spirits were lightened, they began to eat again, and a few were discharged once more. . . .' So we tried to speak to Jane frankly, but she rebuffed our efforts to talk about dying.

Had we misread the signals or had we misread the book? Both, probably. No two human beings respond in exactly the same way. Kübler-Ross had not made it clear enough that the various stages identified in the book need not follow in the strict order in which she described them, and that the various aspects of dying may be present in any of the stages. Each patient is an individual who makes his or her own pattern of dying. We would have been spared worry if we had known this at the start.

We were beginning to concede that there was no hope, and that all we could do was to help Jane to accept her lot. But our attempts were useless without real communication. Painful efforts to reach her were usually less direct than Victor's invitation to get her to talk about dying. The wall of silence was up. But behind it, what was Jane thinking? Did she believe Victor had now given up hope while she was fighting on? Did she feel, What's the point of talking to them?

But if Jane was growing further away from her parents, to others she was becoming closer. Kate, a friend from university days, visited her regularly. Due to go on holiday to Paris, Kate told us later of the day she came to say goodbye. She walked with Jane to the corridor window. There they watched the movement of people and traffic in the street below, comings and goings that seemed to have no purpose at that distance. They were in real harmony, and even smoked a cigarette together, puff for puff. Kate thought this more the kind of thing that lovers did – an action symbolic of closeness and understanding – a one-to-oneness, a statement of intimacy. Kate and Jane had known these periods before, but never had the feeling been so deep and emotional. Jane reached out impulsively to kiss her friend goodbye – and Jane had always been undemonstrative. Kate wondered if that kiss had been merely a farewell on the eve of her holiday departure or whether it was intended as a final goodbye. She went home with a deep unhappiness, a feeling she would never see Jane again. When she reached Paris she spent a long time choosing a postcard and then searching for words that, combined with the picture, would convey something of what she felt. The card never reached Jane. It was lost either in the post or in the network of hospital mail.

Michael's visits were less successful. He brought a friend, Ruth, with him, and it seemed to Rosemary, watching one such encounter, that Jane minded very much. (She was not to reveal her feeling about this until much later.)

The third dose of chemotherapy would be due soon, and we clung to the hope that this time it wouldn't be so bad. Other patients didn't suffer so much, we were told. One woman came for an injection, lay down for an hour, then went home to look after her family. Another woman, who had felt as ill as Jane in the beginning, was soon able to go back to work while still receiving treatment. Research was producing new drugs with less toxic side effects. Only a few years ago, they told Jane, her reaction would probably have been much worse.

She didn't ask us to leave again – at times we thought we could see something like pity in her eyes as she looked at us. The tone of the messages that friends passed on was different now. Yes, we did sometimes make her angry, because our presence reminded her of everything she would lose if she didn't get better. She was coming close to acknowledging that she might have to give up. 'If I do die,' she told James with a laugh, 'I'll miss my rows with Dad.'

It wasn't only her parents who were going to lose her and were mourning the loss in advance. Jane was now anticipating the grief of parting, suffering her own loss of parents, because they would be dead, to her, once she was gone. She worried about what would happen to us – she had been prepared to nurse us when we became ill, to look after us when we grew old. How would we manage if she wasn't there? But these were thoughts she shared with friends, not us.

This new tenderness – or an old tenderness become newly apparent – still alternated with the flashes of anger that had distressed us so much when she first returned to the hospital. Why was she like that, why, we kept asking our friends. The answer that moved us most seemed at first too far-fetched to believe; but the more we thought about it, the more sense it made. She knew how much we loved her, how difficult we would find it to bear her loss. She knew that the more loving she was now, the greater our heartache would be later, the longer it would last. But if she could cut herself off from us, act out fully the anger she was feeling, make us bear the brunt of it, then perhaps we might see her as she really was. And we would grieve less for her.

'What Jane is saying to you is, "Look what a monster I am,"' James told them.

'She tried to make you feel you had failed her, so you'd dislike her,' another friend said.

From the hints Jane dropped, we concluded that this might well be part of the explanation. Jane had been cruel in order to be kind. Perhaps. But she had also been cruel with the selfishness of one hopelessly ill, who cares nothing for the feelings of others. If she knew she was dying, that explained everything and justified everything.

And it seemed as if she finally did know. The knowledge had come to her gradually, even while she denied it. The most the doctors said now was, 'There is no reason to lose hope.' What it seemed to mean was that hope was on the way out – and Jane was aware of it.

Yet the tests had disclosed no new outbreak of the cancer. Jane was still excreting cancer cells in her urine, but that was not unusual after an operation, and the chemotherapy treatment was designed to deal with it. But she felt the cancer was still in her.

'I don't think of it as Big C,' she told James. 'I think of it as lots of little Cs, nibbling away inside like rats in a sack of grain. Or like life growing the wrong way – inward instead of outward.'

James wondered if the time might be right to try to bring her closer to her parents. He suspected that he knew just how bad things were, and he thought they should reach a better understanding before the end, which might come fast. So he told her she had been very bitchy, especially with Victor.

'I know,' she said. 'But that's what I am. There's a bitch in me. I don't want Dad, or Mum, or anyone I'm really close to, to think that I'm better than I am. I believe you have to fight, literally fight, for a close understanding with another person. It's a struggle for the truth, really. I want people to tell me the truth, to respect me that much. Of course, when you're feeling bad, the people close to you are the only ones you really trust with telling how awful you feel, and that's hard on them. When I act like a bitch towards people, it's instead of screaming. I'm not hiding anything. I'm not pretending. If I'm going to die, I want to know.'

When James told us about this conversation, we found it easier to live with Jane's rejection. It was also more difficult to keep the truth from her; but what *was* the truth? Yes, we thought she was going to die, she might even be dying now, but the doctors insisted there was some hope of remission that could give her at least a few more years. 'There is no reason to lose hope,' they kept repeating, as they recalled some of the remissions they had known. There was the man, said one doctor, who had been operated upon but still had a pain afterwards, and continued to excrete cancer cells, and then had a successful course of chemotherapy. He was able to go back to his job driving a London double-decker bus. He came in for checkups, and it wasn't until eight years later that he had to have another operation. 'When we opened him up, he was all black with cancer inside, but he'd had eight years of useful life.' No, they insisted again, so long as they had not found something definite, there was no reason to lose hope. We had been ready to accept that all was over, and then fresh promise seemed to appear, like a mirage.

Jane shared something of the same attitude. At one moment she was telling James that she wanted the whole truth, at another she was saying that she didn't want to give up – having made it clear that even to talk of the possibility of death was to surrender. So James supported her in a feeling of hope. He talked of the fallibility of doctors, of his own recent illness in New York when the doctor hadn't been able to spot his simple hepatitis though his face was yellow. 'A doctor's knowledge is still very sketchy,' he told her. 'The human body is half a mystery.'

'That's how I feel,' said Jane. 'It's very important to think positively and not give up. The mind's control over the body's functions can be so strong. I don't want my body to be cut up. I don't want to be drugged out of my mind. I want my body to have every chance to cope with what's wrong. A plant that's hurt sometimes successfully grows over the wound. So do some animals, like cockroaches. Their bodies can go on with all kinds of growth when they escape from a human attack. I want to give my body a chance.'

But she also talked about how her body had failed her mind, and James felt she might be willing herself to accept that she was going to die soon.

Rosemary still groped for an opening to tell her the truth she seemed to demand.

'How can you bear to go on with so much suffering all the time?' she asked her once. But instead of admitting that she'd given up hope, Jane said: 'Mum, I can remember what it was like before.' There was no answer to this, and Jane showed no desire to talk about it further.

She had always been fastidious. When she hadn't been able to keep herself clean, either the nurses or Rosemary helped her to do so. But now there was nothing visibly wrong with her body, and as far as the nurses could tell, she was able to get up to go to the washroom. They knew about her pain – she'd complained often enough – but it wasn't incapacitating, and they wanted to encourage her to do as much for herself as she could. So they didn't offer to help her wash, and she didn't ask them. When Rosemary offered to do so, Jane curtly declined. When Victor urged her to wash Jane, Rosemary retorted that this wasn't the time to infringe her liberties. She had so few.

So Jane lay there unwashed. She didn't even brush her teeth. The smell embarrassed Victor. One day he apologised to a doctor who had just been examining Jane. 'She's so weak,' he said, 'she can hardly open her mouth to eat, let alone do her teeth.'

'We're used to smell,' the doctor reassured him cheerfully. But he didn't tell the nurses to clean Jane up.

When she made some particularly wounding remark to Victor, he wanted to tell her, 'Jane, your breath smells, do something about it,' but he stopped himself. She always managed to have the last word. When he finally did remark, 'Jane, you're behaving like a bitch,' she smiled at him for the first time in days – a sweet, almost coquettish smile – and said, 'But I *am* a bitch!'

Chapter 6

Jane had now been moved into the farthest corner of the ward where the nurses seldom passed. They would come to administer the painkillers, but only after all the other patients had been taken care of, even if Jane had been ready and crying for a pill long before. They had strict orders that the pills were to be given every two or three hours, so, to be on the safe side, they made it every three. Those who had once joked with her no longer stopped by her bed. They were too busy with other patients for whom they could still do something.

One young specialist used to visit her at the end of the day on his way home. He would ask how she was, would talk sympathetically about her latest symptoms, but it was more a friendly chat than a medical visit. Now even he had stopped coming.

When Jane did manage to talk to a doctor, she tried to question him about her chances, but rarely received any answers. Although no one said anything, Jane was getting the message. The signs meant that she was reaching the end of the road. This certainly wasn't what the doctors wanted to convey to her, but she picked it up from the way they spoke, the way they appeared to have given up. 'What's the point of my staying here,' she asked, 'if they can't do anything for me?'

There were other signals from within her own body that seemed to confirm it. She had been resting for a long time, receiving the appropriate medication and treatment, but she was getting no better. On the contrary, she was growing steadily worse. She could observe her own decline from day to day. She was eating very little. When a doctor felt her stomach, there was a hard ball under his fingers. It was 'probably' constipation, he said. Jane was alert enough to pick up the 'probably'. If it wasn't constipation, it might be another tumour, and she knew what that meant.

That doctor now avoided her. We suspected he was avoiding us, too, so we tried to make an appointment with him. We were told he was away. When would he be back? He wasn't expected until after visiting hours, 'by which time you will be gone.'

'No, we won't,' said Victor firmly. 'We'll wait for him.'

We sat outside the ward to make sure he wouldn't slip past us. He arrived late in the evening, pale and tired, and sat down on the bench beside us. He had had to perform several operations, he said, and then to give a lecture. He seemed to be trying to convince us that he hadn't been avoiding us, and we believed him. Perhaps nobody was ignoring Jane, either. Worry made the imagination do strange things.

He talked to us about the difficulties of the illness and about pain. He was obviously making a real effort to meet us on a human rather than a purely professional level. As he spoke about Jane's illness, he was really telling us how little the medical profession knew about melanoma. The specialists had previously tried to give the impression they knew what they were doing, that they were in command of the situation. But this doctor didn't pretend to be a medical superman. He had no easy answers for us, no reassurance, perhaps not even any hope. In the past our talks with him had been strictly professional, businesslike, but now he spoke of feelings. He told us he understood how we felt because he had a sister suffering from an incurable disease. When he went to see her in the institution where she was being looked after, each journey was one of despair, each visit a nightmare. He, too, asked himself whether nothing more could be done to ease her suffering. 'Believe me,' he said, 'I know how you feel about these bloody doctors.'

Somehow what he was telling us about his sister got entangled with what he was saying about Jane, how everything possible had been done for her, too. She had had the most skilled surgery, the most advanced treatment, the best care. It was almost as if he were trying to justify himself. He spoke of Jane as of an old friend; 'the dear girl,' he kept saying. We asked whether she ought to be told now that she was dying. He rejected the idea as unthinkable. 'No, no, she isn't dying – we have no reason to say so. She's so young – she mustn't . . .'

He was very emotional and very tired, but he tried hard to help us. Yet for all his denials, the impression we got was that Jane was actually much worse, that he felt he had failed and was guilty and distressed. We tried to reassure him, to tell him that the hospital had done all it could, that he personally had been most helpful, kind and supportive, although we hadn't in fact always felt so friendly towards him. He must have realised that he left us with a gloomy conclusion.

Next day he waved to us cheerily, rested, a new man. 'She's a bit better today,' he said. 'She'll have the laugh on us yet, you'll see. I've got a feeling she'll prove us all wrong and still be around half a dozen years from now.'

The effect of this remark on Rosemary was the opposite of what he had intended. *Six more years of this*, she thought bitterly.

At last in May the tenants vacated Dairy Cottage. We packed our belongings with a sense of relief. We got up very early and drove off before breakfast, through almost empty streets, out of London, down the motorway to the country.

The world seemed especially beautiful. We never lost that inner anguish that had been with us so long, but this day it seemed to heighten our awareness of beauty. The house and garden were full of peace. We had come home after a long, hard journey.

But everywhere there were memories of Jane as she had been and never would be again. The nightmare of the past four months had travelled with us. Jane, who should have been there too, eating breakfast with us on the terrace, was imprisoned in a hospital bed. Nothing had changed.

If only she could escape from hospital and come home again, then what little remained of her life would be more tolerable. Surely we would all be able to talk, understand each other, clear up the difficulties and differences of the past weeks?

Two days later the blow fell. Victor phoned Rosemary from the hospital. 'They've got the latest test result,' he said. His voice was heavy, flat. 'It's in the bone marrow.'

This *was* the death sentence. Finally and absolutely. Melanoma cells in the bone marrow meant that there was no hope, no sense even in continuing treatments. There was nothing to be done. Nothing. Jane would have to be told.

'You don't tell a twenty-five year old she's going to die,' one of the doctors admonished Victor. 'It would make her life miserable to the end, and you don't know how long that will be.' 'Believe me,' another said, 'I've had a lot of these youngsters through my hands. I know how they react.' But mightn't Jane be different? Did we want to take the risk? Once she knew, there would be no way to undo the telling. The unhappiness, the non-communication, the rejection – all could get much worse. Would we really be able to cope? Did we even want to try?

The old solution was offered again: take her away on holiday and see how things went. 'Give her a good time.' In the meantime, they could speed up radiation to ease the pain before she left the hospital. Then, if there was a crisis, they would send an ambulance at a moment's notice and bring her back. She would have all the drugs necessary for as long as she needed them. 'She won't know anything . . .'

Not only were the experts prepared to assume the moral responsibility for not telling Jane, they were urging her parents to avoid making the decision, too. 'If she does want to be told, if she can take it, we'll know. We can decide then.'

'That's a decision *we* will make.' Victor suddenly asserted himself. But even as he spoke, he knew he had been persuaded.

Now that the time had come, we were glad to shift the responsibility. The doctors' advice seemed intended to ease our own burden during the period that remained. We could easily imagine how Jane's anguish and resentment, her anger and bitterness, could poison our lives and what remained of her own. If we followed the experts, she might have as peaceful and quiet an end as possible. If we didn't

... Victor in particular was haunted by the image of an incurable invalid, demanding constant attention, blackmailing us emotionally with the knowledge that death was just around the corner. No, better that Jane should *not* know.

But when we called Richard in Boston, he insisted Jane should be told at once that she was going to die. He would fly over within a few days. He would be straight with his sister. 'If you can't tell her,' he said, 'I will.' She had said that if Richard returned, she'd know she was dying. How were we to let her know he was coming? Neither of us could face it.

At the hospital Jane was informed she could go home for the weekend. This was her first chance to see Dairy Cottage since her return to England, but she told us it wasn't worth the pain of the journey. We wondered if she didn't want to be with us.

Then she relented. She told James she might go home the following weekend. To everyone's surprise, she took the news of Richard's impending arrival quite calmly. She spoke of how good it would be to see him again. She appeared to accept that he was coming now because this was a convenient time for him to see her.

James brought Hugh, a mutual friend whose wife had recently died of cancer, to see them. He hoped that hearing Hugh talk of his own experience might help Victor and Rosemary. Hugh stayed for supper in the garden. It was a beautiful evening, with the last rays of the sun golden on the hill beyond the pond. The air was cold and quiet, disturbed only by our voices.

'I want Jane to come home,' said Rosemary. 'I think this would be a far better place to die than in the hospital ward.'

'No doubt about it,' Hugh agreed. 'She should be at home. That's the only place to be.'

'We've been told that young people ought to be in hospital because of symptoms that might be difficult to treat, because there may be sudden crises, or just because it's more distressing when someone so young dies.'

Hugh grunted. 'Nonsense. They said all those things to me, but I brought Catherine home.'

'But how did you manage? You were working . . .'

'I brought nurses in,' he said simply. 'I used to go out and get what they needed, pads for the bed and things like that. Yes. It was the only place for her to be. We shared a bed until the day she died.'

Richard had brought a surprise with him – Arloc, his fiancée's son. At first Rosemary wondered whether Jane's dying was something an eleven-year-old should experience. But Arloc had watched his grandfather die of cancer only two years before, and the boy had coped remarkably well, despite the loss of someone he loved. Richard, at odds with his parents on the question of whether Jane should be told, needed the emotional support of his new family. Joan couldn't come, but he and Arloc were very close. He thought of Arloc as a son, and was sure it would be good for Jane to meet him. He wanted Jane to know all about his new family, in the hope that she would get a sense of continuity, a feeling that children were growing up to take the place of those who left. She had a great sense of nature's cycles and this might console her.

Rosemary had feared that Jane might break down when Richard appeared, but as he walked into the ward, her face lit up with delight. Then she turned to Arloc and asked, 'Who are you?' a little puzzled, only to add with a quick smile, 'Of course, how silly of me . . . Who else could you be but Arloc?' Arloc smiled back at her. 'Good guess,' he said. It was the beginning of a new friendship.

Jane looked better than Richard had expected, but he found the meeting very painful, 'devastating', as he described it later. He could see that she was less optimistic, and she plied him with questions which, if left to himself, he would have answered frankly. But he obeyed his parents' wishes. He didn't lie or give her false hope, though perhaps that was what she wanted to hear from him; instead, he hedged. He had come to help her when she needed help most, and yet he had to play our game of deception, unable to share his feelings with her. He found it very difficult.

In preparing Dairy Cottage for Jane we all tried to forget the family tensions. We were glad to be back with our family doctor again. Dr. Sullivan told us he would do everything possible to help us nurse Jane at home. The district health visitor, who was responsible for organising home assistance as part of the National Health Service, came to see us.

We sat on the terrace, discussing, first, the physical arrangements for Jane's return to Dairy Cottage, and then the family obsession – what Jane should be told. We recounted our differences to the health visitor, a slight, dark-haired woman. She listened carefully to each of us. She agreed with Victor and Rosemary that nobody should force the bad news on Jane. She also concurred with Richard that Jane ought to be told – 'if she wants to know.' Nothing was decided, but we felt much better for having talked in the presence of a sympathetic neutral observer. It was important to settle our differences before Jane came home.

Richard believed strongly that Jane's condition would soon deteriorate so much his mother wouldn't be able to look after her. Rosemary felt equally strongly that home was the only place for her daughter. She wanted no more hospitals, no more strangers in charge. She could remember Jane's weak whisper on one of the bad days: 'Mum, don't let me die here, don't let me die in hospital.'

'Can you imagine what it could mean to have Jane here?' Richard asked. In blunt detail, he described the last stages of brain cancer in Joan's father. 'Mum, please,' he implored Rosemary, 'you must be realistic. Jane will get much worse. You must know that. She'll need expert care round the clock. You'll be exhausted, drained, just when you need all your strength.'

Rosemary's face showed no emotion; it was as if she had hardly heard him. Dairy Cottage, she insisted, had always been a good place to live. It would also be a good place to die. As for looking after her, nurses could be hired if necessary. She asked the health visitor for her opinion. 'Don't you agree that home is the best place?'

Philippa – we were on first name terms by then – agreed there was no better place than home, but stressed that some forms of cancer could take a very difficult course. The National Health Service would provide some free nursing help, and the Marie Curie Society could assign full-time private nurses, day and night, if Jane needed them. They should also bear in mind that if nursing Jane became too difficult, a hospice might be the answer.

A hospice. Rosemary had made enquiries about St. Christopher's Hospice, ages ago, it seemed now, but Jane wasn't interested and they did nothing further about it. To Victor, who was in Washington at the time, this was a new idea. Philippa had to explain that a hospice was not a hospital, but a small unit design for treatment of the terminally ill, mainly cancer patients. How could it help Jane when hospitals couldn't? Philippa told him that patients could go in and out, often staying for a few days, just the time required to get their pain under control. If Jane's pain grew worse – and there was every reason to expect that it would – she could have a short stay in a hospice and then come home again. The staff were good people, she would be well cared for. 'It is not a house of death,' Philippa added. There was a hospice near Oxford, an hour's drive from Dairy Cottage. She suggested we should look at it.

We felt there was still plenty of time; it was hard to believe a hospice could be that much different from a hospital. As Philippa got up to go, she said: 'Do remember now, you're not facing this alone any more. We'll help you all we can.' She left her phone number and promised to visit regularly once a week, more often if necessary.

We continued to argue about whether to tell Jane, but at least she had helped us to be more open with each other. Richard was afraid Jane would begin to distrust him as she had come to distrust us. Perhaps this was already happening. Soon, he feared, she might decide there was *nobody* she could trust, and then she would feel completely alone. We were starting to bend under Richard's unrelenting pressure, but were not yet persuaded. We conceded only that Jane should be told if she made it clear that that was what she wanted. But when Richard said, 'All right, let me ask her,' we wouldn't agree. What else could she say to that but Yes? We managed to discuss everything concerning Jane's future quite dispassionately except this ('They alternate between being very sane and very out of it,' Richard wrote to Joan), and yet a decision would have to be made soon because Jane was coming home at the weekend.

'Let's put the problem to Dr. Sullivan,' Victor finally suggested. Rosemary liked the idea. They knew Richard admired their family doctor's common sense. And he immediately agreed, perhaps convinced that Sullivan would be on his side.

We made an appointment. When the time came, we all went into the little office together to lay our views before him as if he were some kind of arbitrator in a dispute. Richard was direct, uncompromising. 'She should be told the whole truth,' he insisted. Victor was equally uncompromising, 'We can't possibly let her know now. She couldn't take it.' Rosemary also argued that they should wait. 'She rejects any effort at real communication. How can we tell her she's dying?'

'She let's me talk to her,' Richard countered. 'I can tell her.'

'Yes,' Victor said angrily, 'and then you'll go off back to America in a week or two and leave us. You won't be able to talk to her then, and she won't be talking to us. What will her life be like? You were describing the physical difficulties. What about the psychological ones?'

'The psychological difficulties are there precisely because you won't tell her,' Richard retorted. 'You said yourself that she doesn't trust you both now. That's because she can see what's going on, she picks up the signals. Jane is no dummy. She can understand that you don't really want to break the news, that you would find it difficult to face, so even when you offer to talk to her, she says No.'

Dr. Sullivan had been listening with great patience, letting everyone argue without interruption. Now he quietly took charge.

'It may be that she reacts differently to you for the reasons you give, Richard. But it may also be that her reactions change. Perhaps she really didn't want to know at the time your parents offered to tell her.'

'Maybe,' Richard agreed reluctantly. 'But then wouldn't that mean she wants the truth now, to judge from all the signs she's been giving me in her questions?'

'You may well be right,' Dr. Sullivan said. 'We'll be able to find that out when she comes home for good. She'll be more relaxed; it should be easier to talk to her. A??. radiation ought to have lessened her pain by then.'

Rosemary feared that if Jane knew she was dying, she might refuse radiation. We still hoped this treatment would ease the pain and at least delay the spread of the cancer. But we also knew Jane was afraid the radiation would affect her looks, cause her hair to fall out.

'The kind of radiation she's being given shouldn't have that effect,' Dr. Sullivan explained. 'But if she does refuse it, it would mean a lot of pain in the weeks to come, unnecessary pain.'

'Jane has been asking me what the radiation is for, what it will do to her. What should I tell her?' Richard asked.

'Perhaps you should leave it to me,' said Dr. Sullivan calmly. 'I can explain to her, and that'll let you off the hook.'

'What do you propose to tell her?'

'That radiation does work well, but also that nobody can be sure it will clear it up. And that's the truth. So she won't be too disappointed if she gets no better.'

'And if she gets worse?' Richard persisted.

'I'll warn her explicitly that the cancer may crop up again. Then, after two or three weeks, if the pain is still there, I can tell her this means the radiation didn't work. There'll be no lies, Richard.'

'And you'll tell her she's dying?'

'Certainly, if it's clear that she wants me to.'

'That's agreed, then, doctor,' Victor said quickly. 'Richard will be back in the States by then. He can trust you, even if he thinks we won't have the guts to go through with it.'

It was a peace offering; but Richard wasn't so easily reassured. 'What are we going to tell her about the bone marrow?' he demanded. 'That's something else she keeps asking me. I think she should be told the result of the test.'

'The hospital said No,' Victor objected. 'If we tell her, there'll be hell to pay when she goes back to hospital. They'll say we're interfering with the treatment. They'll wash their hands of her.'

Dr. Sullivan assured Victor he was wrong about that. But he agreed with Richard that Jane should be told the result of the bone marrow test. He would do this himself, he promised.

'You will?'

'I don't think you ought to doubt Dr. Sullivan's word,' Rosemary said, embarrassed.

'Well, I think I ought to be there when you talk to her.'

'Richard, really!' Victor cried angrily.

'That's quite all right,' Dr. Sullivan said gently. 'There's no reason why Richard shouldn't be there.'

It was small comfort for Richard, but better than nothing. He felt he had let Jane down. He wrote to Joan: 'I feel such a failure for not pushing more successfully that Jane should be told everything.'

Meanwhile, Jane's own questions at the hospital were becoming more persistent. When she asked a doctor about the result of the bone marrow test, he assured her there was no evidence of cancer in the bone. That was what he'd agreed with her parents to say. He told her playfully, 'You already know too much, Jane.' To Jane, this meant that she couldn't trust him, that he must be keeping something from her, and she could guess what.

'The doctor says Jane is withdrawing,' Richard told his mother when he came home from visiting her in London. And he added bitterly: 'I wonder why.'

Rosemary didn't reply. She wanted no more arguments. She was putting all her faith now in getting Jane home to Dairy Cottage.

Chapter 7

Jane's return coincided with the start of a long holiday week-end, part of the British Royal Jubilee celebration. The Queen was to light a huge bonfire in the grounds of Windsor Castle, which was only a few miles from Dairy Cottage. It would be the signal for thousands of bonfires to be lit throughout the country. On the patch of common land at the end of the lane near Dairy Cottage a towering pile of wood had been collected in readiness. Perhaps Jane would feel well enough to watch the flames. She had always loved a bonfire.

Victor went to the hospital earlier in the day to check that she was ready. The rest of the family were sitting on the terrace when we heard a noise from Victor's room. He had gone upstairs to change without even telling us he was home. When he joined us, he was obviously making an effort to appear normal.

'You're back early,' Rosemary said carefully. 'Is anything wrong?'

'No, nothing's wrong.' He sounded angry.

'I don't believe you.'

'All right, then,' he burst out suddenly. 'It was a disaster. Jane threw me out. She screamed at me, the little bitch. Everyone in the ward could hear!'

They absorbed this in silence. Then Richard asked, 'Do you think she'll come home tonight?'

'Frankly, just at this moment I don't particularly care.'

Rosemary tried to soothe him. 'It must have been rough. You shouldn't have been on your own.'

Victor looked down to the pond where Arloc was playing in the boat. 'Don't worry, I'll get over it,' he said.

The sunny afternoon passed slowly. We heard nothing from Jane, although she was physically capable of making her way to the phone in the hall. If she felt too ill, she could have asked one of the other patients to call.

Friends had offered to drive her home in the evening while we were busy with last-minute preparations for her return, but by nine o'clock there was still no Jane and no news. It was getting dark when at last we heard the sound of a car in the drive. We rushed to the door to see Jane coming slowly down the garden path ahead of her friends. She was wearing her bright Indian waistcoat and smiling cheerfully. Although she was obviously tired, she didn't look desperately ill. There was colour and life in her face, almost a brightness. She held up a small bottle. 'Tanya gave me this for the journey,' she said with a laugh. 'She says vodka helps her when she's in pain.' She kissed us all, including Victor, as if nothing had happened. Her outburst at the hospital seemed trivial. All that mattered was that Jane had come home.

The journey and the excitement had wearied her, and she was soon ready for bed in the little room at the end of the house on the ground floor. It was quiet there, far away from the noises of the rest of the house, and next to a bathroom. There would be no stairs to climb, she would feel close to the garden – her bed was pulled right up against one of the windows.

'You've made the room look lovely, Mum,' she exclaimed. There were flowers on the table by her bed, flowers on the desk beside her woven baskets and wooden boxes, flowers on the windowsill beside her. Thick rugs lay on the floor and heavy curtains, striped in the earthy colours she loved, hung at the windows. 'I never saw before what a beautiful room this is,' she said, looking round at everything and then staring out at the dark woods for a few moments before settling back on her pillows with a sigh of relief. She was soon asleep that night.

The next morning Jane dressed and tried hard to be a normal member of the family. She went into the dining room for breakfast with the rest of us, but even a soft folding chair proved too uncomfortable. She retreated to the sitting room sofa, but was unable to arrange her limbs without discomfort. She tried to use her stereo, but could lift only one record at a time from the pile and had difficulty finding what she wanted. Rosemary offered to help her. At first Jane wouldn't say what she was looking for. Only when it was clear that the search was proving too difficult did she admit that she had been trying to find Fauré's *Requiem. She thought it might upset me*, flashed through Rosemary's mind as she put the record on. But it was Jane who couldn't listen for long. 'Switch it off,' she said. 'It's too sad.'

Just before noon the person we had all been waiting for – Julian Sullivan – arrived. He talked to Jane alone. Richard no longer insisted on being present. We waited on the terrace with Jo, a friend who had come to cut Jane's hair. It proved to be a long wait. We sat in silence much of the time, wondering what was being said. At last the doctor came out alone to join us.

He said quietly, 'She was ready, so I told her. She accepted it easily.'

We all had the same question: How long?

He could only venture a guess – maybe six months.

There was nothing more to be said. He left quickly so we could go to Jane.

We found her on the sofa, crying a little but in control of the despair she must have felt. One by one, we kissed her and she returned our embraces, weeping but not breaking down. There was no drama, no great climax to the months of uncertainty, of family argument and friction.

Victor asked what the doctor had told her.

'He said I should expect less rather than more time. Now every day will be a bonus.' Her voice was calm, as calm as the doctor's had been.

She made it sound so simple, so direct; but it hadn't been quite like that, as Dr. Sullivan told us later. He had led the conversation carefully, letting her ask the questions and giving her the kind of answers that would encourage her to probe more deeply if she wanted to – or to avoid the issue. 'We walked our way around it,' he said. 'I was trying to feel her out, leaving it to her to ask, "Tell me more." '

He knew she was worried about the radiation, and

explained that the radiotherapy was treating the spread of the disease in her bone in an attempt to relieve the pain. He was being optimistic. But if she listened carefully, she would hear that his expectations were strictly limited, that he was promising only an alleviation of her symptoms, no more. Jane picked up every nuance, and pressed him to be more direct. For once she was not preoccupied with the pain.

'How do I know if it's doing me any good? If it's worth having?'

He realised that he could take it a little further, be more specific. They expected to ease her pain, he repeated, but no one really knew how well the treatment would work. If the radiation did bring relief, that would be a sign that the cancer cells were being killed off. 'At least some of them,' he added, almost as an afterthought. 'The most active ones . . .'

'And if the pain continues?'

Now he knew they were on thin ice. He had in fact anticipated this question, and already answered it, at least by implication. So he could be even more direct. 'If it doesn't work, then we'll wonder if it has done any good.'

He still wasn't taking away all hope, and he never would. Now that they understood each other, they no longer beat about the bush.

'We both knew that we were talking about dying,' he told us. 'Neither of us had used the word, and I had made sure that I'd left her a thread of hope, the possibility that the treatment *might* do some good. In my mind I knew that there was no such thread, but if she wanted to cling to hope, she could. Instead, she made it clear that she wanted to be realistic, and we no longer needed to walk around it.'

He felt her relief, and now he could share in it. With this clarity between them, she could restate her question and be sure of a clear answer.

'If the pain comes back, what am I to expect?'

Dr. Sullivan felt she was asking him how long she had, and he replied immediately, almost abruptly, because this was not the time for evasion. That was when he told her, 'You'd probably have six months,' and left, so that Jane and the family might at last share the truth, and the grief, in private.

But having accepted death, Jane turned back to life.

'We'll try to make it as good a time for you as we can,' Rosemary said. Other promises had been broken in the course of her illness. Rosemary hoped she would be able to keep this one.

Jane glanced at Jo, who had withdrawn into the background. 'Will you cut my hair now? It looks so foul and I'd like to be respectable again.' She gave precise instructions, knowing that her friend would do what she wanted. 'Very short,' she said. 'It looks so straggly. It badly needs a wash, too.' She seemed to be doing her best to avoid an emotional scene. The rest of us watched in silence as the haircutting started and the two friends began to gossip as if it were an ordinary day. Jane laughed as Jo described her children's antics. The tension eased a little and slowly we all relaxed. It was clear that Jane wasn't going to pieces. Now we could be completely frank with her and live whatever time she had left in truth.

Richard went to Arloc in the garden to tell him that Jane now knew she was dying. The boy's reaction was matter-of-fact. 'She knew already,' he said. No, he hadn't talked about it with her. 'It was something that was there.'

When Jane's haircut was finished to her satisfaction, she said, 'Now that I know I haven't got much time left, I want to enjoy every day, and I'd like you to help me. For a start,' she added, 'let's go round the garden.'

Arloc fetched her stick and we set off on a tour. At first Jane walked with her arm through Rosemary's, but when they reached the terrace she took it away. She rested her weight deliberately on her stick, testing the extent of her independence. It worked. Then, very slowly, she dragged herself round the garden. She walked carefully, head down, watching for obstacles or uneven ground that might upset her precarious balance.

She must have worked it all out for herself. It couldn't have been an instant, instinctive reaction to what the doctor had told her – this calm, this acceptance. She had often thought in past months of the possibility of dying. She must have decided that when she knew for certain, she would face it, accept it, and extract what happiness she could from the remainder of her life. Did she also realise how much she would share that happiness with others?

Jane appeared quite unworried during that walk, aware only of the beauty of the garden. She stopped at the edge of the pond and stood for a long time leaning on her stick. The surface was covered by a solid green carpet of duckweed that cut off the life-giving light from the water beneath. We wondered what she was thinking as she stared into the dead pond.

Then she walked through the part of the garden she had always lingered over, through the old avenue of yew trees that stopped short at the fence. Those trees must have been planted for some special purpose, perhaps to make a grand entrance to a long dead house. There was a carpet of yew needles beneath the darkness of the branches where no plants grew and no rain penetrated. Jane walked very slowly, her head always down. To see anything above ground level, she had to stop and steady herself before looking up. This dry place beneath the old trees was full of memories for her – evening picnics by a fire, building and firing primitive kilns for simple pots, times of solitude and times of companionship. Part of her life had been spent here. It was as if she were drawing strength from these memories. Or was she saying goodbye?

'If you have the energy, you shouldn't miss a particularly fine rose by the French windows,' Rosemary said gently.

The rose had opened from its first tight red bud and was at its most beautiful, Jane put her nose close to it.

'That's certainly a five-star rose,' she said.

She had a brief rest and then took part in a tree-planting ceremony. She had got Richard and Arloc to buy her a Victoria plum tree for Rosemary's birthday and they had dug a deep hole beside the stump of a cherry tree. They had put peat in the bottom, then Arloc brought the hose and soaked it with water. By the time Jane made her slow, careful way up the garden path, all was ready. She leaned heavily on her stick while the plum tree was planted and the soil shovelled in, then watched as the rest of us trampled it down. When the slight young tree had been tied to its supporting stake, Victor opened a bottle of champagne. We drank a ceremonial toast – to the tree and to Jane.

Before going back into the house, she took a last look at the garden, as if she realised she was seeing it for the last time.

We found it surprisingly easy to talk to her, as if all barriers had been removed. To Richard, she confided that she'd known everyone was stringing her along. She'd minded at the time, but it was over now. She harboured no ill-will, she had no reproaches for anyone. When Rosemary pressed her not to return to the hospital, she said: No, she must go back and finish the radiation. It did seem to be easing her pain somewhat.

'Oh, Jane. That awful chemotherapy you went through, all those treatments. If only we'd known what was going to happen, you could have been spared so much misery.'

'Don't worry, Mum,' she said. 'If I hadn't had them, I'd never have known whether they might not have cured me.' Her words were comforting, but the tone of her voice, the expression on her face, said much more. Once again she could cope with what was happening to her.

They could see the jubilee bonfires glowing in the sky, but the celebrations seemed irrelevant. Jane lay in bed, too tired to visit the local bonfire.

Four days later, she went back to the hospital. In one hand she carried Tanya's bottle of vodka, refilled, in the other a letter written by Victor to the doctor who had urged them not to tell Jane what was happening. Victor made it clear that Jane now knew she was dying and that the family wanted her to leave the hospital as soon as her radiation treatment was over.

At the hospital our decision was accepted without any discussion. Jane was told that the treatment, which had been planned to extend over two to three weeks, would now be compressed into three days. But they didn't speak to her about what she knew; the taboo remained in force.

Richard and Rosemary went to the hospital to bring Jane home on a day of torrential rain. The roads were choked with traffic, and visibility was down to a few yards. They dreaded the return journey under such conditions, knowing that every bump in the road would hurt her.

The hospital, as always, was briskly anonymous, but Jane was cheerful when Rosemary arrived for her. She had somehow managed to get on most of her clothes unaided. She'd also assembled her few belongings from the locker and was now lying back, exhausted. Rosemary pulled on Jane's socks and long boots. They were both keen to escape as quickly as possible.

Walking proved difficult, even with a stick and Rosemary's support. 'No wheelchair,' Jane said firmly. She said goodbye to the other patients as they passed through the ward. 'I must say goodbye to the staff, especially the nurses.' Earlier the ward had been full of doctors and nurses, busy with the morning routine, but now none were to be seen. When they reached the passage, they found that, too, was empty. Nor were there any nurses in the other ward. This was rare.

'I did want to see them,' Jane said. They shuffled laboriously back and Jane asked the other patients to make her farewells. 'Tell them I'd like to have thanked them for all they did for me,' she said. Then she leaned on Rosemary and moved slowly towards the exit. She didn't say anything on the way out, but she looked upset. Later she told us why: not a single nurse had come to say goodbye. They all knew she was leaving the hospital that day. Perhaps they hadn't been able to face her, especially as she now knew the truth.

Richard brought the car as close to the entrance as possible. We helped her into the back seat, already piled with cushions and rugs. She leaned back and closed her eyes.

'I'll try to drive round the bumps, Jane,' said Richard, easing into the driving seat.

'Don't worry, Rich, I'm really comfortable.'

Suddenly all the difficulties and delays seemed to be behind them. The traffic was light, the rain eased off and the sky lightened. Richard drove with great care and Jane did not complain. She lay with her eyes closed until the car pulled up before Dairy Cottage. Then she opened them and said: 'That's the easiest drive I've had since my shoulders got bad. Thanks.'

The first morning she talked of getting up. 'But I feel so weak,' she said, 'so worn out . . .' She stayed in bed and slept a lot. We thought it was the journey that had worn her out, but the next day she was again too exhausted to leave her bed.

'It's the radiation,' Rosemary told her. 'You're bound to feel tired after such a big dose. You'll be better tomorrow.'

She didn't feel better the following day, but in spite of her exhaustion, it was a good time. She was glad to be home. When she said she was happy, it was easy to believe it. Her face reflected the pleasure she took in being alive; her calm manner and affectionate ways seemed to show her inner contentment. The sense that we might be losing her soon made the experience of the present far richer, even when we shared tears.

Jane could talk to her family again, to each member separately or to all together. The estrangement from her parents was in the past. Her relationship with each of us was a different experience, and her reactions to us varied accordingly. She might smile tolerantly at parental density or obstinacy, but there were no rows now, no cold silences.

We talked again about the possibility of her going into the hospice at some future time, but each of us felt differently on the issue. Richard insisted she should be admitted as soon as possible; Rosemary wasn't convinced that Jane would be happy there; and Victor, pulled between them, wavered and changed his mind from day to day. Jane would agree with each in turn. She needed to feel close to us all and could not risk being isolated from any one.

Richard was perhaps the most relieved. He felt that his long struggle had been vindicated by Jane's easy acceptance of the truth. Rosemary was reassured because her early attitude to Jane's possible suicide was also vindicated by a conversation her daughter reported. Jane said she'd raised the subject of an overdose with Dr. Sullivan. He'd looked at her seriously and told her: 'If you do that, Jane, then I shall know that I have failed you.'

She now knew that her painkillers wouldn't be rationed. This doctor wouldn't expect her to be stoic and endure, but would help her all he could. Secure in this trust, Jane never spoke of taking her own life again.

We planned for a long time ahead. It was the second week in June, and Dr. Sullivan said she might still be with us at Christmas. Richard helped organise the house so that Rosemary would have the minimum of work to do. We bought labour-saving gadgets and a capacious deep freeze which we filled with food. There would be no worry about preparing meals. Jane's friends could be properly fed when they came to see her. Richard and Arloc went to Infinity in Brighton to obtain special vegetarian foods. The staff there took the trouble to help and also sent a large present of apple juice, which became Jane's standard drink.

Arloc was a frequent visitor to Jane's room. He came and went when he felt like it, sometimes settling to talk for a long time, sometimes just popping in and out. He was the moving spirit behind the construction and maintenance of a bird table outside her window. Victor helped with the basic structure, but the boy added many improvements as the days went by. Jane watched the procession of bird life with joy and fascination for hours on end. She was concerned that the small birds should get their share without being driven away by larger birds or squirrels, so improvised food containers were strung from a nearby tree. The squirrels were particularly clever, and Arloc worked hard to keep one step ahead of them, although it was their cunning in reaching the apparently unreachable that gave Jane the most pleasure. Soon it became difficult to meet the demand. Arloc put out all the left-overs, then robbed the pantry for nuts and raisins. A failed batch of bread was a feast one day, beans from a broken jar were soaked until soft and put out for a special treat the next. Jane enjoyed herself, forgetting all the claustrophobic months in hospital. 'Look,' she would exclaim, 'a greenfinch . . . a sparrow.'

Arloc helped install an elaborate intercom system so that Jane could call if she needed help or company. The wires trailed through the house, round pictures, over door frames. We fixed an extension in the pottery so that, when Jane had settled down, Rosemary would be able to work with an easy mind knowing she could be summoned if necessary.

In the hospital Jane had been given a pepper plant by

one of her friends, and she said she would have liked to feel that she had a garden of her own growing. We installed a vegetable garden in peat bags outside the sitting room window where she could see it. The plant was joined by tomatoes and runner beans. Once again Jane had a garden of her own.

Rosemary wished she didn't have to spend so much time on chores, but the house wouldn't run itself. She knew Victor and Jane needed time together, and between mother and daughter there was no unfinished business. Yet no human relationship is ever as full as it could be, and when time is short, it is heartbreaking to feel that any of it is wasted. None of us knew how little time Jane had left.

Chapter 8

Apart from the pain, one obstacle remained to Jane's peace of mind. Richard was the first to sense the undercurrent of anxiety beneath her outward calm, and he helped to bring it out into the open. She told him of her anger over some of the things her father had said and done as much as ten years earlier, when she was still a child. Richard urged her to have it out with Victor. But how could she, without making him feel guilty? This wasn't what she wanted to leave him with when she was gone. Her love for Victor made her suppress these bitter, angry memories, but Richard realised she needed to get them out to be completely at peace.

'My next task,' he wrote to Joan, 'is to try to get them talking really honestly with each other. This may well be impossible. I cannot afford to take the risk.'

Yet when he mentioned it to Victor, delicately at first, ready to pull back at the first hint of trouble, he found that his father was more than willing to talk to Jane about some of their past disagreements. He felt none of the guilt, he said somewhat aggressively, that Richard expected him to wallow in. They had been honest disagreements, and he had sought to act fairly by Jane. 'Maybe you've read too much Freud, but I didn't do anything I need to feel guilty about, so I don't.'

'Bullshit,' Richard exploded. Then he added more gently, 'Dad, one always feels guilty about people one loves.'

Richard's intervention worked. Victor agreed that it was time to clear up past differences, and their talk stimulated him to examine his memories – and his conscience. He remembered when Jane was fifteen and he had taken her on a trip round the world. They had flown from Tokyo to San Francisco, seen the sights of the city, then returned to the airport for a flight to Washington, DC. Jane's physical exhaustion soon translated itself into one of her 'off' moods. At first she was silent, but he would not let her remain so, for he thought he recognised the warning signals. He tried to get her to talk again by involving her in the preparations for the departure, asking questions she would have to answer; but she became angrily uncommunicative, only grunting in reply and deliberately averting her face in a way that seemed calculated to attract the attention of the other travellers.

It made him squirm. She had displayed these moods before: in Israel, after a tour of the battlefronts of the 1967 war which had been fought a couple of months before; in India, after walking through streets which had become homes for the poor, the ill, the hungry; in Hong Kong, where they lost their way in what looked like an anthill teaming with millions of frantic human beings. But she had usually managed to keep her feelings to herself. Now she was making a public spectacle of them and showing that very lack of self-control he had hoped the trip might cure. When she was in this kind of state, there was no reaching her; but he had to make her realise what she was doing to him and to herself, how she was destroying the good their trip had done, how she must learn to live with herself, with others. At that moment nothing seemed more important to Victor than to shock Jane out of the state of sullen rebellion she had sunk into, a state so characteristic of her behaviour before they set out on the trip.

Inside the airplane, Jane appeared to be having some difficulty with her seat belt.

'Here, let me help you,' Victor said, as he reached over to her.

'Can't you leave me alone,' she almost shouted.

That did it. He snapped: 'If you insist on behaving like this, Jane, you'll never make any friends. You'll go through life on your own. And if you make any, you'll never keep them.'

She looked at him without a word, then turned her face

to the window. Watching out of the corner of his eye, Victor saw a solitary tear roll down her cheek.

They didn't speak of the incident, but after they got back to England, Jane told her mother about it, and Rosemary attacked him furiously. 'What a terrible thing to say! She's insecure enough as it is. She'll never forget it. She'll never forgive you.'

And she never did. It was one of the things, Richard said to his father, that remained to be sorted out. But Jane would not mention it herself.

Victor looked for ways to raise the subject. Several times he was on the point of speaking to her, then each time drew back. At last he said, without any preliminaries: 'About that day in San Francisco . . .'

Immediately she knew what he was talking about, and tried to make it easy for him to go on: 'Yes, Dad, I suppose we were both pretty beastly.'

At once he was on the defensive again. 'Well, Jane, I didn't mean to be beastly. I thought I was trying to help you.' He went on to explain his motives. He really had been concerned about her future, how she would be able to make friends, build a life of her own.

Jane didn't pull her punches. 'That hurt a lot, Dad. It still hurts. I'm angry whenever I think of it.'

'I'm sorry, Jane. What else can I say?'

But an apology was the last thing she wanted. 'Well, do you still think you were right?'

Now he knew what else he could say. He spoke of the friends she had made at the university, of the young men she had loved and who loved her in return, of the children who became devoted to her when she taught them. 'Of course I know I was wrong. But I didn't know it then.'

That seemed to be all Jane required by way of an admission. She didn't want to make him feel guilty, and she even helped a little by talking of her own prickly behaviour as a teenager. 'I know I must have tried your patience.'

In the days that followed, they spoke of other incidents and problems left over from those times. The human misery Jane had witnessed in Asia had strengthened her radical tendencies, and on her return to England she became increasingly active in the political movements of the late sixties, flirting with Communist and Maoist ideas. At home she would put all the passion of a sixteen year old into political arguments with her father which usually started calmly enough but rarely ended without acrimony. He thought he was paying her a compliment by treating her as his intellectual equal, answering each argument with a counter-argument of his own and requiring her to back her assertions with evidence. At least that's what he told Rosemary when she pleaded with him to go easy on Jane. But he could easily produce the evidence to support his own arguments, and he gave no quarter when Jane faltered in debate.

Jane's arguments were what one would expect from an idealistic teenager – passionate, intense, earnest. He pursued every remark she made in the heat of the moment to its logical conclusion and proved its absurdity, to his own satisfaction. When Jane spoke of injustice and suffering and pain in a world that Victor too knew to be far from perfect, he sometimes recalled his own youthful dreams of righting the world and tried to tell her he understood what she felt; she would grow out of it as he had done, because things were not as simple as they seemed. In reply she would rage and storm at him for betraying his own ideals and would swear to stand by hers, come what may. His aim was to convince her that some of her ideas were impractical, and while conceding that a few might be feasible, to show her she was going the wrong way about gaining support for them. Her aim was to demonstrate to him that the world was in a mess and that he was one of the people responsible for it. She didn't care whether he thought her ideas were right; she knew they were. She wouldn't be argued out of them, as he had argued himself out of his own ideas when he was her age. She wouldn't betray her ideals as he had betrayed his. He was trying to remake her in his own image, but she would not allow it, never, whatever the bribe – and she threw the round-the-world trip back in his face.

Richard, two years her senior, was then at Harvard, deeply involved in the Vietnam War opposition and student protest movements. His relations with Victor remained good, perhaps because he was away from home, and he too advised his father to go easy on Jane. 'Let her win some of the arguments,' he wrote. 'She is insecure. She needs to think she is right.'

But it was too late. Jane no longer talked about politics with her father, and if he tried to raise the subject, she wouldn't respond. When they spoke of other things, it was clear that there was a barrier between them. The old intimacy and the new passion of their recent debates had gone out of their relationship. Both were on their best behaviour – or tried to be, because they knew that further argument might completely destroy a relationship already gravely damaged, and they wanted to avoid that. The stand-off continued for more than a year.

Their relationship began to grow warmer again only when Jane left home to go to the university. It took her another year to become disillusioned with student politics, and then with politics generally, but she never changed her view of the world, never lost the feeling that injustice was the condition in which most of mankind lived, never shed the burden of guilt she had acquired when she saw the real world during that trip with her father.

Since then, they had never talked about their old disagreements, or acknowledged that either might have been at fault. When Victor now spoke of it, at Richard's urging, the anger Jane showed at the recollection of their quarrels was so quick he wondered whether he might have done better to have kept silent. She had forgiven him easily, graciously, for the San Francisco incident, but she was still bitter about the way he had browbeaten her intellectually when he should have known she was not mature enough to compete with him in a political argument. What had hurt Jane most of all was Victor's opinion of her motives. Her recollection of their arguments differed from his. She felt that he had accused her of favouring violent solutions for the world's ills, of caring more for her theories and political preconceptions than for the people whose cause she claimed to espouse. He had questioned her honesty, ridiculed her values.

Victor was appalled at the picture she had carried in her mind all these years. He could see now why their reconciliation had never seemed complete, why it had lacked the depth and warmth he longed for. Had he really been so insensitive? At first he thought of assuring her that it had not been his intention to treat her in this way, that she must have misunderstood him. But would that be true, and was it even relevant? More important was that he now knew her values had been right, that she had been honest and sincere, and that he could assure her of this without the slightest qualm.

Victor didn't limit himself to empty assurances. He talked to her of that day in India when she came back to their plush hotel so sickened by the poverty she had seen in the streets that she couldn't get a morsel of food down.

'But you made me eat, don't you remember?' she interrupted him.

'What I remember is our discussion. You were so upset that you wouldn't go out into the street for several days and then, when you did go, you were so angry when you came back that we had another row.'

She had returned to the hotel in a fury and treated him to a detailed description of the poverty and misery she had seen that day. She followed it up with a scorching attack on a capitalist system that allowed things like that to happen. She didn't attempt to analyse the system or propose a cure for its ills. 'You're the political expert,' she mocked.

Then she listened sceptically as he propounded his solution – a world in which the United States, Russia, and China would join forces with Europe and Japan to help the rest of humanity gain a tolerable standard of living. International co-operation between the advanced countries to help those less generously endowed would take the place of the arms race, and a golden age would bring to the whole of mankind the benefits individual nations and civilisations had sometimes enjoyed during their own golden ages.

'Rubbish,' she exploded. 'Did you ever stop to think of the slaves during the golden age of Rome? Or of the disease and hunger and poverty of the common people during the Renaissance?'

'They didn't have modern technology,' Victor replied feebly.

'You mean like the technology they're using in Vietnam?' Jane scoffed.

He spoke of swords being turned into ploughshares, while she accused him of mouthing platitudes. Why, she asked, if he really cared about the people they had seen in the streets and villages of India, had he not written about the problems of the under-developed countries? That wasn't his area, Victor countered. 'But who knows, perhaps I will. Yes, I think I should.'

She relented. 'Is it a promise?'

'Yes.'

It was Jane who reminded him, as they reminisced at Dairy Cottage about this conversation they had ten years ago, of the promise he had made to her, and he reminded her, in turn, of some of the articles he had written on the subject since then. 'I don't think I would have written them if it hadn't been for you. I'm glad, now, that you went for me.' It was out of character for Victor to speak in this way; he wasn't usually contrite. But he didn't want her to think he was just saying this because he knew she was dying. 'I really mean it, Jane.'

'Did you mean it about the golden age?'

'Of course I did.'

'You haven't written about *that*.'

The time hadn't come for it yet, he told her. No one would take him seriously if he did. Sooner or later . . .

'That's what you said in New Delhi, Dad. You told me things were moving in that direction, that it would happen in a dozen or two years, and if not, then in a score or two. Don't you remember?'

'No.'

'And there was something else you said, Dad.' She was deliberately trying to jog his memory.

'What, Jane?'

'You said, "I may not live to see it, but you will." '

There was an awkward pause before Victor answered: 'No, I don't remember that, either.'

'Well, it doesn't look like I'll outlive you now, does it?'

His distress must have shown on his face.

'Don't worry, Dad. I think I can take it. And if I can, then you can, too. I've had plenty of time to get used to it. That's what I was thinking about most of the time in hospital.

That's when it was hard. That's when I couldn't talk to you.'

'It's all right, Jane, it's all right now,' he repeated mechanically, as one does to a child who has been hurt. 'It's all right.'

'It was hard on you, too, I know.' She wasn't apologising so much as explaining. But with those few words she wiped away the hurt and anguish he still felt when he remembered the weeks of rejection.

It was true that he *hadn't* felt guilty, as he told Richard. It was also true that, as Richard had feared, there was a risk in making Jane and Victor speak about the past because now he did feel guilty about it. But it was a guilt he could live with. It was only because she had been able to talk to him that he could sit by her bed silently, look into her eyes without averting his own, and discuss the other thing that needed to be talked about when a person is dying – death itself.

He said he doubted whether many people would have reacted to what Dr. Sullivan had told her the way she had. 'I know I wouldn't.' How was it she was able to accept it without protest, so quietly, so naturally?

'Because it *is* natural,' she replied.

Victor didn't think it was, not for someone her age, but he stopped himself from saying so aloud. Instead, he asked: 'What do you mean, "natural"?'

'There are two ways you can look at it, I suppose. In a geographical sense, and a historical one.'

'You do have a philosophy, then?'

'I don't know if you'd call it that. I used to think when I was in hospital, in the geographical sense, look at me lying in this bed, in this precise place on earth – me, Jane, in a city of seven million – and every day, every hour, every minute maybe, somebody is dying here in London. And London's in England – fifty million people, all of whom are going to die, sooner or later. And England is only a tiny part of the world, with four billion people, which means that there must be millions dying all the time, all over the world, thousands at this very moment. In this geographical sense, what am I but a speck? What's the earth but a speck? Why should my dying be so unacceptable and so difficult to bear? Why should it be more unacceptable than theirs? What's so special about me?'

'And the historical?' Victor prompted.

'Well, look at the world and how long it's lasted, not just civilisation, but humankind. Look at the millions and billions who've come before us and died, year after year, century after century, for thousands and thousands of years – and all the billions who'll come after us, and will die. Obviously, this is something that *is* happening, that *has* to happen, so why not accept it? Why resent it? Why fight it? It has to be. It is. And that's all there is to it.'

'It's logical enough. But the fact is that I am afraid of death, and you aren't.'

'I was afraid all right, at first. But I've had plenty of time to think of it. All these months. I knew my chances were pretty low. There were times when I said to myself, I'd rather die quickly, now, than go on like this. And there were times when I was prepared to try anything, put up with the worst that the chemotherapy or radiation could do – the vomiting, the convulsions, my hair falling out, anything, so long as there was a chance. The fear was worst at night. In the daytime, with people around me, it was easy to be calm. At night, when everybody had gone, when I was alone, I'd be so exhausted that I longed to sleep, to forget. But I couldn't. As soon as I tried to sleep, the fear got too big. The only thing I could think of was all these cancer cells whizzing around my body, or worse still, finding new places to grow, spreading inside my body, dividing, growing, taking over. Eating away at the healthy parts.'

It was the first time Jane had spoken to him so directly about dying, and she had done it, he now realised, only after he had told her of his own fears. It was almost as if she was trying to help him overcome his apprehension. She wasn't succeeding, but he was determined not to reveal that. He dredged up another memory he had long suppressed.

'I think I know how you felt. Do you remember when the doctor first told me I had angina? I came home and we sat on the terrace as the sun was going down, and it took me some time before I could bring myself to tell you and Mum what he had said, and you were both so kind and loving and reassuring. I just sat there and couldn't say anything much.'

'You took it pretty well, Dad. I remember all right. Perhaps that's where I get it from.'

Did she really think he took it well, or was she still trying to help him? Perhaps that was how it had looked to her. But to him the doctor's verdict was like a sentence of death, the threat of a heart attack that could come out of nowhere at any moment. He had faced the thought of death much as one might look directly at the blazing sun for a moment, and then averted his eyes from it. It blinded him. It wasn't something he could contemplate. Feel, yes; think about, no. But what he felt was the sense of non-existence, a vast emptiness, an abyss of nothingness. That's what's called ego-chill, he had thought to himself as he shuddered with fright – and put it out of his mind.

Only now, at Jane's prompting, was he beginning to think of it again, reluctantly, for one thought led to another, and sometimes he would find himself reliving his wartime nightmares. Jane's questions showed that she knew what was going through his mind, and she tried to get him to talk of his experiences in the war. He knew she was trying to help, but he could not respond. He wasn't ready yet.

During this week friends from London came to sit by her bed, talk about old times, hold her hand, and cook her favourite vegetarian dishes. They knew what Dr. Sullivan had said, but Jane's calm acceptance of it and her obvious happiness at having them there made these days good.

She was anxious that everyone she cared for should have something of hers to remember her by – something that would please them and be useful. She began to match possessions and friends. Books, pots, household treasures, all the things she had chosen with care and bought from her earnings or received as gifts, would now become part of the lives of the people she loved. Sometimes she asked Rosemary to buy a special present when she had nothing appropriate to give someone. With Rosemary's help, she made lists of who should get what. 'It's giving you such a lot to do,' she apologised. 'This is something I really ought to do for myself.' But in this time of easy understanding and communication, Rosemary was able to reply. 'It's simpler to do it all now, while you're here with us. If I leave it until you've gone I may not be able to cope – it'll hurt much more then.'

They sometimes cried together about the inevitable parting. Rosemary would tell Jane of the many reasons why she would never forget her, remind her of the memories that would keep her alive. Jane had been an important part of all their lives; how could she cease to matter to them? Love wouldn't end when her body died, in that sense she wouldn't be dead. She'd still be around. How could the things they'd learned from Jane ever be forgotten? She would leave so much behind her, not only memories but things made with her hands, practical things that could be used and enjoyed, beautiful things that could be looked at.

'Yet it is so hard to lose you,' Rosemary told her. 'There's a poem by a Russian woman, Anna Akhmatova, whose husband and son were both carried off to the prison camps: "This must be happening to someone else. I could not have borne it." That's just how I feel. But I have to bear it and I know I will.'

Once or twice Jane mentioned her hope that her parents might adopt a child – some deprived youngster, underprivileged, perhaps from the developing world.

Jane and Rosemary had talked of death in the early days of her illness as something inevitable but impossible to imagine. Rosemary had told her then of a dream she'd had. 'It was extraordinarily happy, and very vivid. I was dead and had been buried under the path by the front door – not the place I'd have chosen. It was just sunshine and warmth on the stones and I was there. It was a very happy dream.' Then Rosemary had still been able to say to her with a laugh: 'When I die, please walk carefully over that bit of path, just in case!' Now she couldn't make that joke. She knew Jane would never tread that path and would be the first to die.

But when Jane talked of death it was realistically, of something soon to take place.

'When I die,' she said suddenly, 'I don't want to be

buried.' Her voice was unemotional; she might have been discussing a haircut or a choice of dress. The disposal of her body seemed a small matter. 'I've always had a horror of being buried alive,' she went on. 'It was one of my nightmares. Will you fix it so I'm cremated?'

'Of course. Lots of people have fears like that. It's very common. Shall we scatter your ashes in the garden?'

'Mmm. Over the pond, too, and by the stream.' She leaned back on the pillow and closed her eyes. They could both hear the rustle of the stream in the quiet evening.

She began to tire more easily. A system of signals was arranged between Jane and her family: One buzz on the intercom meant she needed something, two buzzes indicated she was tired and wanted to have a visitor tactfully taken away. The buzzer was carefully hidden under the covers so no one's feelings would be hurt. Whoever answered the call was not to let on that they had come in reply to a summons, but to make it appear they'd just dropped in. However, she never used the two-buzz signal.

As the pain increased, the possibility of Jane's getting up became more remote. Soon she couldn't visit the bathroom next door without help. The next day, when she asked Rosemary to help her, she could barely put one foot in front of the other. She had to force her legs to make the steps. Her feet splayed out under the weight of a body unable to obey the mind's signals. To sit down on the toilet seat was an additional misery. She crouched on the lavatory with Rosemary struggling to hold her upright and cried: 'What am I doing to you?'

Rosemary half-carried her tortured body back to the bed that seemed to give so little comfort. She knew now that Jane should never attempt to get out of her bed again – she should struggle no longer. She phoned Dr. Sullivan, and barely twenty minutes later he was in Jane's room. 'We'll get help for you,' he said. 'You needn't try to manage alone.' The district nurses were on their way. They would make her bed, wash her, lend her a bedpan.

To the rest of us, he said, 'She should go into the hospice as soon as possible. I'll see if we can get the paperwork done quickly.' The decision was made; there was no more discussion. It was obviously the only thing to be done. 'The cancer is moving so fast we can hardly keep up,' Dr. Sullivan said. The hospice had more applications than it could cope with, and for every patient it admitted, several were turned away. But he knew that Jane's youth, the rapid deterioration of her condition, and the intensity of her pain would all give her priority.

Rosemary had no more arguments. It was gradually becoming clear to her that it would be impossible, even with full-time nursing help, to look after Jane at Dairy Cottage. She clung to the hope that, after a week or two of treatment in the hospice, her daughter would come home again. When the time of death was near, she must be surrounded by her family's love.

'She keeps complaining about her feet,' Rosemary told the doctor. 'Sometimes she says they're hot, sometimes cold. Then she'll ask us to rub them. And she'll say, "I can't feel — are they hot or cold?" '

He met her eyes sadly. 'It's the beginning of paralysis. There's nothing I can do about it.'

Jane was finally trapped by her disease. Trapped and helpless. She lay in bed by the window barely moving, her head turned towards the bird table, her eyes following the movement of the birds. When she lay still, the pain didn't bother her much and she was calm and relaxed.

When Dr. Murray, the consultant in charge of the hospice, heard the facts of Jane's case from Dr. Sullivan, his answer was instantaneous. She was in terrible pain and needed help immediately; he knew the hospice could provide that help. She could be admitted straight away.

Adjusting to their diminishing expectation that Jane might still have some life worth living left to her, Victor and Richard went to inspect the hospice.

Jane and her mother waited peacefully for the men to return — it wasn't really waiting, just a shared time together. They watched the restless activity round the bird table outside the window as birds settled, fed nervously, then fluttered away. The weak constantly gave way to the strong, to return when their chance came again.

They didn't talk much, just a few words here and there.

'You know, I really am happy, Mum,' she said. 'I'm in pain, but it doesn't matter, I'm happy, do believe that.'

The house was very quiet.

Victor and Richard burst in with a rush. Their exuberance was so intense it was as if everything in the peaceful room jumped. 'The hospice is a marvellous place, Jane,' Victor said. 'Just wait until you see it. It's not a bit like a hospital, more like an ordinary house.'

Richard put in, 'The doctor is really a terrific man and the nurses are superb. They all talked to us – really talked with us and not at us.'

'They're getting a single room ready for you,' Victor went on happily. 'There's a bird table outside the window. What's more, there's a visitors' room so we can even stay the night.'

Jane and Rosemary exchanged looks that said, There they go again, so easily carried away. Aloud, Jane said: 'I think it's time for my medicine.' She could still joke at her own expense. 'Judging by the sound of my voice, it's past time!'

When she was alone with Victor, Rosemary asked what the hospice was really like; but his enthusiasm was sincere. 'The man in charge is sure he can get her pain under control, although it may take a little time. He wanted to know all about Jane – I described how the hospital doctors wouldn't let us tell her she was going to die and he was completely on our side. I'm absolutely convinced we're doing the right thing. They would have admitted her this evening if we wanted, but if we wait until tomorrow she can go straight into a room of her own.' He handed her some papers. 'Here's a list of things we should take.'

Rosemary ran her eye down the list. ' "We'll be waiting to welcome you," they say. That's a good beginning.' She read on aloud: ' "Nightgown, brush, comb, hand-mirror, etc. Day clothes" – well, she won't need them. Nor will she need notepaper and pen, slippers, dressing gown . . .' She stopped again.

'They were most insistent that we should bring those things,' he said. 'They try very hard to make the patients feel at home. It's warm and comfortable. There's a lot of modern equipment to make things easier for the staff . . .'

'More machines?' Rosemary shivered, remembering the huge, mysterious monsters she'd often watched being pushed down the hospital corridors. She'd found it impossible to guess whether their purpose was to clean the hospital or perform some operation on the patients.

'No machines. If the patients need treatment or therapy, they're taken to the hospital next door. But the hospice is quite separate, it really does look like a home – curtains, carpets, pictures.' He told her it had been built to a modern design, with the comfort of the patients as top priority. Only twelve of the twenty-five beds were in use. The funds were not available to staff the others.

Victor had informed himself about the hospice background with his usual thoroughness before deciding to entrust his daughter to it. This hospice had been established with private funds, some donated by the National Society for Cancer Relief and the rest raised locally. But once built, it had been handed over to the government-funded National Health Service to be run as part of the system open to all who need medical attention, free of cost. We were fortunate to live relatively close to it. There were only about half a dozen such units in the United Kingdom, and Dairy Cottage was just outside its official catchment area; but Dr. Murray was free to stretch a point when he felt the situation demanded it, in spite of red tape. Private hospices like St. Christopher's are completely independent and usually separate from hospitals, but the units funded by the National Society for Cancer Relief are built in the grounds of already established hospitals, can use the full range of their services, and are always in a position to return a patient to the main part of the hospital if further palliative treatment should be required. Although the area health authority which takes over a completed hospice is responsible for staffing, administration, and running costs, it manages the hospice in keeping with an operational policy previously agreed between the National Society for Cancer Relief and the local authority. In this way the specially trained hospice doctor who is in charge retains the autonomy he needs to run his establishment on principles which may sometimes seem at odds with generally accepted notions of what a hospital is for.

Victor's explanations satisfied Rosemary, and she had managed to relax a little when a new problem presented itself.

Late in the evening Jane needed the bedpan. In happier times, the pan the district nurses had brought would have amused the family considerably. It was a large, upright model, with gothic lettering round the rim solemnly proclaiming that the patient would be more comfortable if the rim was covered with warm flannel. Modern bedpans can be slipped under a recumbent patient, but not this one: Jane had to sit upright. It took a joint effort by Rosemary and Victor to lift her into position. Every movement hurt her. She sat on it awkwardly as they both held her up, one on each side, the pain showing in her face. They waited. 'I can't pee, Mum. It won't come.' She struggled on, but in the end she had to give up and we laid her down in bed again. Then, driven by her discomfort and a growing fear that she would never be rid of all the liquid pressing inside her, we tried again. This time Victor wedged his back against hers so that she could lean on him and not depend on her own diminishing strength to sit upright. He wanted desperately to help her and at the same time was afraid that every movement he made could hurt.

She cried out with pain and frustration and quickly begged to be laid down again.

It was now that Rosemary realised fully how utterly impossible it would be to look after her. How could they nurse her when every touch on her body caused pain? How could they even move her, untrained as they were?

The immediate need was to get relief from the pressure in Jane's bladder, and to free her mind of the fear that she'd never manage to pass water – a fear that was rapidly developing into panic.

Dr. Sullivan was out that evening, going to three meetings one after the other. Jane pulled herself together again. 'Let's have one more try,' she insisted. Miraculously, it worked. Tired out, we began to settle for the night.

Jane's fingers were too weak to press the buzzer. All day

her only pleasurable physical contact had been the feeling of a hand beneath her own. Whoever sat with her would slip a strong, healthy hand under her weak fingers to give her the human touch she longed for.

Rosemary made up a bed for herself in her daughter's room. Jane was given her late night dose of medicines and sleeping pills. Exhausted, they settled to sleep.

Victor's voice came out of the darkness, his head round the door. 'Are you asleep, Jane?'

'I was, almost.'

'The doctor's here, he wants to know if you're all right?'

'Fantastic man!' she murmured, still half asleep. 'Tell him I'm all right.'

A few minutes later Victor was back. 'He says he'll sleep better for knowing that.'

'I think I will, too,' she said.

The next morning the pain was worse. A district nurse arrived early intending to give her a thorough wash, but could only sponge her face. When she heard of Jane's latest difficulty, the nurse was reassuring. 'Don't worry about the waterworks, dear. They'll give you a catheter – they slide a little tube into you and you won't have to bother any more. The liquid will just drain out, it won't hurt at all.'

Punctually at nine Dr. Sullivan arrived to give Jane an injection to enable her to endure the journey. He brought a bottle of medicine to top up the injection. 'One or two spoonfuls as often as you need it.'

There was no sense of haste about his visit. He sat beside Jane and she gave him a goodbye present. She tried to thank him – so did we – but there were no words to convey what his help had meant to us.

Rosemary needed reassurance about the hospice. 'You do want to go there, don't you?' she asked. 'We're not forcing you into something you don't want to do?' She leaned low over Jane's bed to hear her answer; it obviously hurt her to talk now.

'It seems the only thing to do. I can't go on like this . . .' The weak voice tailed away into silence.

It was already past nine, the time the ambulance had been expected. We were beginning to feel anxious, but Jane remained calm. Her face was composed and her manner detached as she lay unmoving, asking nothing except an occasional spoonful of the medicine. Time passed slowly. As tension in the family rose, Jane gave the appearance of being in a world apart. She was obviously in pain, but she didn't complain or express anxiety about what lay ahead. She was unable or unwilling to be distraetd by conversation. She lay silent, staring upwards.

At last a car door banged at the top of the path and Richard came running in from the garden. 'They're here!'

As the ambulance men carried her gently out of the house wrapped in a red blanket, up the steep path, the younger man fumbling at what was obviously a new job to him, the birds were still singing, but she gave no sign of hearing them now. It was just a week since she had walked down this path on her return from hospital.

What does a father think when his twenty-five-year-old daughter is being carried off to a home for the dying? This father thought, with a shudder, that she would never see her home again – and that she would be much better off at the hospice than at home. What does a mother think? This mother thought that the most terrible moment of all had come, and she was overcome by a sense of failure – conviction that she had failed to preserve the child she had given life to and nurtured for so many years.

The ambulance journey was a nightmare. With every jolt, every grimace, it was as if a knife was being driven into Jane, deeper every time. The younger man drove very slowly, very carefully. The older man stood up in the back with us, watching Jane's face, repeatedly telling the driver to go more gently, trying to make bright conversation to distract her, while his eyes reflected the pain and desperation communicated at every jolt.

In contrast to our small world of pain, outside was pleasant, easy country, the kind of scenery Jane would have loved when she was well. Freshly cut fields of hay were scattered between fir plantations and small villages lay in the hollows. Sheets of white daisies reached over the grassy slopes each side of the road. We passed an ancient cottage with an old cart wheel attached to the chimney stack. Here in this cottage, Rosemary thought, people had grown old and died over a long period of time, generation after generation. Jane would never grow old . . .

At first we tried to behave as if there was no need for hurry, but the injection was wearing off. The ambulance man decided to drive faster, yet the pain was now so intense that the remainder of the journey was a torture to Jane. When at last we reached the hospice, the older attendant told us, 'We'll just go and see what's happening,' and disappeared. Jane spoke into the silence that followed. 'Just another bloody hospital after all,' she said clearly.

The two men returning swiftly from their reconnaissance had an answer for her. 'You've got it all laid on here, Jane.' The older attendant's voice was free of tension at last. 'You must be someone special. Your bed is made up, the doors are all open, you go straight in – no messing about at all!' She tried to smile back at him.

We were outside a small, low building, modern in design but unpretentious. This was in a far corner of what was a general hospital area, on the edge of the countryside, and very quiet. The only vehicles that travelled the little road were those coming to the hospice. Nearby were huts built during World War II and since converted for general use as clinics and offices, with signs showing their function. But in the hospice, all the patients' windows looked out over a view of green fields and trees. It was as if the hospice were quite separate, an oasis of calm which gave no hint of the busy hospital life.

It was only a few steps to the front door. Quickly, efficiently, without a wasted movement, the two attendants wheeled Jane's stretcher bed from the ambulance into the hospice. The nightmare journey was over.

Chapter 9

A young woman was waiting with a smile just inside the door of the hospice. 'Hello. I'm Elizabeth Jones, one of the sisters here. I've come to get you settled into your room.'

As the two attendants wheeled the stretcher along a cheerful, carpeted corridor, Sister Elizabeth walked beside Jane, talking to her, trying to make her feel at home. 'She's the one who showed us round yesterday,' Victor whispered to Rosemary.

Richard and Arloc came hurrying to meet us. They'd gone ahead to help get Jane's room ready. 'We thought you'd never make it. We've been here for ages,' Arloc said. 'We've had a good look round. It's a terrific place!'

'Hello.' Another nurse came up to us. She was tall and vigorous-looking, with a welcoming smile. 'My name's Patricia. Would you all like some coffee, or would you prefer something stronger after that journey?'

Things were falling into place. We were at the hospice, we had been expected and, it seemed, were welcome. We still inhabited a world of pain, but we were no longer isolated in it. We sank wearily into armchairs in the lounge.

'Would you help me to fill in this form about Jane, please?' The hospital secretary sat down beside Rosemary. This was the first time that Jane hadn't been able to speak for herself, but the questions were the usual ones. Rosemary paused for a moment over 'Religion?' and then answered as Jane would have done: 'None.' She remembered Jane's first experience when she had had the black spot removed, and how upset and angry she'd been when a receptionist snapped that she'd no right to be a teacher if she wasn't religious.

'People like that shouldn't be in such jobs,' Jane had said, wiping away tears of tension and anger.

A wild thought now crossed Rosemary's mind: would they refuse admission to an atheist? But the secretary showed no reaction.

The atmosphere of the hospice was very informal, almost low-key. It was more like coming to a friend's home than an institution. In Jane's room all was ready. The porter brought in a vase of flowers and put it where the new patient could see the blooms most easily – 'something lovely for her eyes to rest on,' he was to say later, when we got to know him.

'This is your new room,' Elizabeth said to Jane. 'I'll get someone to help us lift you up on to the bed.' She was back in a few minutes with Emily, another sister. Working together with the help of the ambulance men, they lifted Jane without upsetting her too much.

'That's a beautiful shawl, Jane. I love the colours.' Elizabeth fingered the crocheted woollen shawl that Jane had worn on so many happier occasions.

With an effort, Jane answered, 'I made it myself ages ago.'

'Now I'm going to give you an injection for the pain,' said Elizabeth. 'Just a little prick, and then the pain will soon begin to ease. Did you feel that?'

'Hardly at all,' Jane said.

'I'll get one of the nurses to put in a catheter for you, so you needn't worry about bedpans any more. Then we'll be back to settle you down.'

'Thank you, thank you.' Jane closed her eyes, relieved that the discomfort of a full bladder would soon be ended.

Elizabeth and Emily, both experienced and highly qualified, were confident that Jane's acute pain would be brought under control fairly quickly. Of the increasing grades of pain – from mild through moderate, severe, very severe, incapacitating to overwhelming – Jane had reached the last stage: the point where consciousness is pain. They could see that she was near to death, and they knew it is harder to nurse the young, who often have greater difficulty adjusting to dying than older patients. That was one reason why Jane had been put in a room of her own, rather than in one of the five-bedded wards. Goodbyes are harder for the young. She would need privacy and the opportunity to talk to friends and relatives.

Both sisters had been warned by Dr. Murray that Jane was likely to prove a difficult case. They knew she should be moved as little as possible. While they set about making her as comfortable as they could, they were also checking for signs of the troubles that beset the bedridden: bedsores, rashes.

At the same time they were taking stock of Jane's physical and mental reactions to every movement and to what was said to her. They wanted to get to know her as quickly and intimately as they could. The more she trusted them and relaxed, the more effective their help would be.

Jane was washed with the minimum of disturbance. The nurses worked to find the most comfortable position for her back and her limbs. The pain she was enduring was so-called superficial pain – that is, pain that fills the body and is exacerbated by the slightest touch, and not deep pain, which is in the bone and is aggravated more by movement. Some kinds of pain can be lessened by laying a patient on a water-bed or on a net, but the nurses decided that Jane's agony could not be alleviated in this fashion. It took about ten minutes before her body had been settled to their satisfaction – and to Jane's. She rested, supported in a nest of pillows, grateful for the relief they had brought her.

Elizabeth picked up the shawl from the chair. 'Shall we put this over the bed? It'll cheer the room up no end.' She waited for Jane to agree, and only then did the two sisters place the shawl over the bed so that its bright colours hid the plain white sheet. They were careful not to give Jane the impression that she was being bossed about. As far as possible, the patient must remain the master of the situation. 'And this little shawl your brother brought with him – would you like it over your shoulders?' Emily asked. 'It's chilly today, really cool for June.' Gently she laid the garment over Jane's shoulders, aware that while most patients appreciated any physical contact, for Jane the lightest touch was painful.

As they chatted with Jane easily and casually, both sisters were also studying her responses to determine whether she needed the help of the hospice psychologist. They decided there was no such need. Jane would have been comforted if she had known this. In the past few weeks she had sometimes wondered whether her mind was failing her.

A thin, slightly stooping, elderly man with a quiet, reserved manner came in. He was one of the doctors. Dr. Murray, the senior consultant, was away until evening and Jane, whose pain was now getting worse, was very disappointed. She felt that this man, Dougal Brown, examined her in a rather cursory way. In fact, we learned later, he had been anxious to avoid causing her unnecessary suffering by carrying out a more detailed examination. He had seldom seen a patient in such distress and he barely touched her. Dr. Murray would examine her thoroughly later. Jane should have been reassured by his visit, but by now everything was irritating her. She asked him, 'Can't you stop the pain? Can't you do something?'

Dr. Brown did not lie. 'We'll do the best we can to help you.'

She needed desperately to feel that help was available, but it was impossible for her to have confidence until the pain began to diminish. Dr. Brown gave her some morphine.

We took turns sitting with Jane. Patricia, the tall nurse who had greeted us in the hall, came in, and her health and vitality seemed to fill the room.

'Hello!' she cried brightly. Jane winced slightly. 'I've come to see if I can do anything for you.'

Acutely sensitive now to his daughter's reactions, Victor responded for her: 'What really matters is that she has proper vegetarian food – *really* vegetarian. She won't eat fish or eggs, and she gets her protein from beans and cheese.'

'Oh, we're quite used to diets,' Patricia said confidently.

'The other hospitals never gave her food she liked.'

A cross mutter came from the bed: 'Always cheese and lettuce . . .'

'I'll see to it. I'll ring the kitchen right now.' Patricia went out.

'Thanks for getting rid of her, Dad. Her voice went through my head. But the pain's still bad. Can you tell them?'

Victor found Patricia outside. Her smile was bright and helpful. She had been prepared for a difficult evening; new patients often took time to settle down and it was only natural that a parent should be anxious. 'I'll ring the kitchen,' she said in a soothing way.

'No, no.' His voice was sharp with tension. 'This is more important. Find Sister. Jane needs another injection.' Patricia herself had full authority to administer drugs, but she said merely, 'All right, I'll tell Sister.' She went to the injection book and was appalled by what she saw. The doses Jane had been given since her arrival were already very high, higher than she would care to be responsible for. But Elizabeth, when told of Jane's request, merely nodded. 'Don't worry, Pat. I'll see to it.'

When Elizabeth gave Jane the injection, she took the opportunity to tell her more about the hospice. Jane confided to her how lonely she had sometimes felt in the hospital. Here, Elizabeth assured her, there would always be company when she needed it. Jane was worried that she might not be able to summon help. The pain in her arms would make it difficult for her to reach the bell. Elizabeth fixed the bell-push so that it would be within easy reach, suspending it from the lamp fixture just next to Jane's head. But Jane still insisted it would be no use to her. 'I shan't be able to reach it,' she said gloomily. What she was really saying, as we realised later, was that she didn't want to be left alone.

When Patricia returned to Jane's room, Victor was holding a glass for her to drink from.

'Here, let me do that for you,' she offered.

'No,' Victor said sharply, anxious to protect his daughter from a nurse she seemed to dislike, 'Jane likes me to do things for her.' Patricia retreated, once more rebuffed. 'I've just rung the kitchen and her diet has been sorted out.'

Victor cut in, 'We can go shopping – her friends can go – we can cook what she wants. Beans, for example. Are they getting her beans? That's what she must have. Beans.'

'I'll check.' Patricia escaped to the comparative calm of the nurses' desk and picked up the phone. This time the kitchen staff weren't quite so polite. Victor reappeared.

'Jane is still in pain,' he said accusingly. 'Can you give her something?'

'The injection hasn't had time to work yet, give it at least half an hour.' Half an hour seemed to him like a lifetime. Fortunately more help came.

The door opened quietly and a small, plump, middle-aged woman appeared. She was dark-haired, with an olive skin and deep, dark eyes. 'Hello, Jane, my name is Adela,' she said, with just a slight touch of a foreign accent. 'How are you feeling?'

Jane liked the sound of her voice, and answered with a smile. Adela had a way of approaching new patients as if they were old and dear friends. Her warmth drew an immediate response, and soon they were talking, Adela's hand under hers. 'Your mouth looks dry, love,' Adela said. 'I'll just clean it for you, shall I?'

She dipped a swab in a pink liquid and then gently inserted it between Jane's lips, working it from side to side. In all her months of illness, when her mouth was often dry, sometimes foul-tasting, no one had ever done this for her. And yet it was so simple, so obvious, Rosemary thought, as she observed Jane's delight at this new procedure. Adela carefully wiped the inside of Jane's mouth with the swab. 'How does it feel, all right?' she asked.

'It's delicious,' Jane said, 'clean, fresh. Thank you, Adela.'

Patricia, who returned just then, didn't think that Adela was doing it properly, as she told us later, but she wouldn't say so outright. Hospice nurses are as careful of the feelings of the junior staff as they are of the patients'. Instead, she said: 'Shall I help you, Adela?'

To Victor, who felt he ought to be protecting Jane from contact with Patricia, this was a danger signal. He put his hand on her arm as she approached the bed and virtually moved her aside. 'Jane wants Adela to do that,' he said brusquely.

Patricia retreated to the nurses' desk, aware now of Victor's hostility. Why has this man taken such an enormous dislike to me? she asked herself. It must be anxiety, she decided. As she was drawing up an injection of Valium for Jane, she told Emily about Victor's behaviour.

'I think that what Jane really needs is not Valium, but a little rest from her father. It's he who really needs this injection . . .' She carried the needle back into Jane's room, and when she went past Victor (as she told us with a laugh later) just managed to restrain a powerful impulse to jab it into him.

Hearing of Jane's distress, Emily wanted to see if there was anything she could do to help. But continual action in the sick room conveyed an atmosphere of crisis. A new patient could be bewildered by too many unfamiliar faces. This was why those nurses whose presence was not specifically needed deliberately kept out of sight at first, introducing themselves only gradually. Emily felt a terrible disappointment, a sense of failure, that the hospice had been unable to help Jane in the first few hours after her arrival.

By about five o'clock in the afternoon Jane's distress began to overwhelm her. She refused to swallow any more medicine. Dr. Brown and Elizabeth stood by helplessly as she spat out the mixture they had given her. 'It's no good,' she cried angrily. 'I won't take it. Why can't I have the stuff I had before?' She wanted the familiar taste of the medicine which had given her some relief during the ambulance journey.

'This is the mixture you brought with you,' Elizabeth assured her, but her concern and encouragement didn't get through to Jane, who was crying bitterly. 'It isn't, it isn't,' she wept, trying to turn her head away, but unable to do so because of the pain. 'I wish I were at home. I feel horrible, everything keeps coming and going away again . . . I hate it here . . .'

'Wait,' said Dr. Brown. 'I'll get the bottle so you can see that we're giving you the medicine you want.' He soon returned with the bottle, now wiped shining clean, and an empty medicine glass. He poured a dose and offered it to her. This time she drank it without a word.

It didn't help much. Dr. Brown, who was comparatively new to hospice work, gave Jane as much morphine as he thought safe – and that was a great deal. Elizabeth, who had been a hospice nurse and sister for many years, thought that Jane should have been given a more powerful dose right from the start. Later everybody agreed that this should have been done, and they freely admitted to us they had made a mistake.

That first evening Jane's room was a sick room. The curtains had been pulled across the window, but the semi-darkness, the painkillers, the Valium did little to help Jane relax. She did not sleep. Adela, whom she already liked and trusted, had gone off duty, and so had Elizabeth. Patricia was now in charge. Dr. Murray, who had given Victor so much hope the day before, hadn't yet returned. Rosemary, Richard and Arloc had gone back to Dairy Cottage for the night, leaving her father alone with Jane.

Victor was anxious and uncertain. Would this be yet another of those endless vigils when we waited in hospitals for doctors who never came or, if they did, brushed past us with a preoccupied air and a meaningless word of comfort?

Jane stirred uneasily. She opened her eyes and said angrily: 'I wish I could get to sleep. Will that doctor of yours ever come?'

Victor wondered guiltily if he had built up her hopes about Dr. Murray and the hospice too much. Her irritation worried him. We had led Jane to believe that Dr. Murray would help her out of the pain, but where was he when she needed him? She was again showing the displacement anger we had first noticed in hospital. Usually patients are careful not to direct this at the doctor on whom they depend for treatment, but Jane seemed past caring.

Victor would have been content if she had chosen him as a target again, for she obviously needed an outlet of some kind to take her mind off the pain. The quiet, understanding talks at Dairy Cottage already seemed far away, yet he was determined that she should regain the repose lost when the pain began to overwhelm her. She must die in peace. This was the whole point of bringing her to the hospice.

Soon, he told her, things would be as they had been at home, and better. He spoke to her quietly, trying to reassure her. There was still so much to talk about, he said, so much to remember . . . But Jane didn't want to speak about dying. She looked at him with exasperation. 'All this talk, talk, talk. Where does it get us? If only they could do something about the pain! Can they? Can they?' she repeated persistently.

It was bound to take a little time, he told her. They had to try different things before they knew what would work. But Jane had heard too many such assurances. Her pain was the only reality. It was here, it was now, while death had once again been dismissed from her conscious thoughts although it overshadowed everything she said.

'What time is it?' she murmured.

'Getting on for seven o'clock, I suppose. I don't know exactly.'

'Does this mean you'll be going home soon?'

He looked at her, startled. Did she want to get rid of him? Was she withdrawing again?

'What would you like me to do, Jane?'

'I know you said they'd look after me here,' she began. 'I'm sure they will. You said you can visit me at any time you want to, no visiting hours.' She spoke slowly, as if she'd thought out what she wanted to say and was trying to find the best way to put it. 'They're good about visitors here, not like the hospitals, aren't they?'

'Yes, Jane, you can set your own visiting hours.' Victor remembered how she had dismissed us from the hospital.

'People can stay as long as they like?'

'All day, if you want.'

'And night?' Now it poured out, what she really wanted. 'The nights, the nights, they're so long, so horrible. The nightmares – the thoughts. I used to get so scared, all alone. I used to think I might die, all alone.' Her voice quickened. 'I don't want to be left alone. Promise me I won't be. Promise me.'

'Jane, you won't be, you won't be,' he said, bending over her closely. She might not want to talk about dying, not now, not to him, but he was sure she was thinking of it. 'They said one of us could stay here. There's a bedroom for relatives. I'll go and see about it straight away.'

'No. Dad, don't go. I have the horrors – don't leave me, ever.'

'What, never?' he said with a smile, using a line from a Gilbert and Sullivan operetta that had become a family joke.

'No, never,' she answered promptly, the fear huge in her eyes.

He held her hand very lightly, felt how cool it was, and wished he could transmit the warmth of his own body into hers. Then he gave her a solemn promise.

'Mum or I will always be with you, Jane. Or Richard, while he's here, or Arloc. If we have to go out, we'll ask one of the nurses to sit with you until we get back. You'll never be left alone.'

His promise brought Jane great relief; but her pain went on.

Now that she had made it clear she wanted him to sleep next to her rather than in the guestroom, he asked Patricia if it could be arranged. She must check, she said. They would have to find a bed to fit in the small space. She wasn't committing herself. Patricia wanted to make sure this was really something Jane desired, and not merely an over-anxious father's idea.

Jane was never left alone again. With someone always in the room, she was free to think her thoughts without the need to deal with others. It was physical loneliness that she feared, the possibility that her body would suddenly erupt into a crisis demanding outside help when no one was there. The assurance that someone was constantly at hand would contribute much to her peace of mind in the days to come. Even that night it seemed to ease her mind until the pain claimed her again.

'Isn't it time they gave me something for the pain? It's getting worse.'

'Let me see if I can catch a nurse,' Victor said. There was no one outside. Should he go looking for a nurse, having just promised never to leave her alone?

'Maybe we should ring your bell?' he said.

'Don't overdo it, Dad,' The edge was back in her voice. 'You can go and find the nurse. I don't think we should ring the bell, they must have plenty to do without that.'

He found Patricia at the medicine cupboard, carefully measuring a milky liquid into a small glass drop by drop, entirely concentrated on her task. He looked around, but saw no other nurses.

He interrupted her. 'Jane is in terrible pain. What on earth can be done?'

'But she's only just had the medicine. We must give it a chance to work.' She looked up and, seeing the anxiety in his face, added: 'I'll come in a moment.'

When Patricia arrived, Jane lay with half-closed eyes, pretending to be asleep. She didn't want to talk to Patricia or acknowledge her presence. The nurse moved close to the bed, studied Jane's seemingly relaxed face, and smiled encouragingly at Victor. She was hardly out of the room when Jane opened her eyes. 'Why didn't she give me something?'

Victor went out again, but Patricia was nowhere to be seen. There was a murmur from the nurses' office. He stood in front of the door listening, recognised Patricia's voice and raised his hand to knock, then suspended it in mid-air.

'Thank goodness you're here,' Patricia was saying. 'Jane hasn't settled down very well, her father is most terribly anxious. We've given her everything Dougal prescribed, but her father won't believe the pain has eased.'

Victor rushed back to Jane's room. 'He's here, Jane!' he almost shouted. 'Dr. Murray's arrived!'

Dr. Murray talked to Jane in her room while Victor waited outside, taut and nervous. He had to wait a long time before the doctor came out. His manner was calm and controlled. He might have been a priest rather than a doctor. Tall and loose-limbed, he led the way to the nurses' office, which was now empty. His movements were relaxed, his speech deliberate, his manner thoughtful. Just now, it seemed, the most important thing was to put Victor at his ease.

'I've had a good talk with Jane and she's in bad shape, but I told her we should be able to do something about it. Her condition is really much the same as before, but the ambulance journey shook her up considerably and greatly increased the pain.'

'But that was at noon. It's seven o'clock now!'

'Yes, we ought to have been able to deal with it by now, but it isn't always so easy. The patient becomes increasingly anxious in such circumstances, and this in turn makes the pain worse.' There was a very intricate mechanism at work here, he explained, a direct relationship between physical pain and anxiety. Fear and the expectation of pain can greatly increase a patient's suffering.

'I told Jane that I'd give her some strong stuff to try to get her to sleep, and that I'd look in later. She said she'd like you to stay, and you're very welcome to – your presence here is very much part of her treatment.'

With a start, Victor realised that Jane was alone, that he was already breaking his promise to her. 'I must get back to her,' he said almost curtly. He could talk to Dr. Murray later.

Jane's pain seemed to have increased in spite of all the diamorphine – another word for heroin – ordered by Dr. Murray. Victor was aware that too much diamorphine could 'depress the respiration', as one book had put it. Jane might stop breathing. And that, he thought, might be just as well. Perhaps she had suffered enough. But it would be a bad way for her to die – in anger and pain. He felt isolated and afraid.

Patricia was also deeply concerned, but she at least was able to share the load of tension and anxiety by talking to Julia, the nursing officer in charge of staff. Julia, who was taking over the night shift, wanted to know everything.

'We're probably going to have a really tough time, not with Jane, but because of her family,' Patricia told her. 'Her father – he kept coming out, asking, "Where's the sister?" as if I wasn't capable.'

'He probably thinks they're still in a hospital and only the sister in charge can make decisions. It'll take the family a bit of time to understand that it's different here.'

'I feel he has no confidence, and we need the family's support to look after Jane properly.'

Julia studied the chart with its story of continually increased doses of drugs. She could understand why Victor was anxious.

'If only we could get the family out of the way, just for a few hours,' Patricia went on. 'You know how patients can put up a show for relatives? I came in and Jane moved her arm. She made a face, but it wasn't a face of pain – just that her arm was stiff. Her father said immediately: "You see, she's in pain. She needs another injection." '

'Did you tell David?' The staff were on first name terms with Dr. Murray, as with each other.

'He just said: "I understand the situation." '

'He did warn us there'd be problems. She was a social science student before she became a teacher, and her father told David she doesn't hold with authoritarian ways. At her last hospital she was very hostile to some of the doctors. David said we should be ready in case her resentment rubbed off on us.'

'Another thing,' Patricia continued, 'she's been given such enormous doses of diamorphine. I keep thinking she's had too much . . . Is it morally right?'

Patricia was wondering whether the drugs might not shorten Jane's life. Julia, with her greater experience, was able to reassure her. 'David knows what he's doing,' she said.

'I never imagined we'd give her as much as this. I told David what I thought and he said we were going to bang it in, bang it in, and get her free from pain before decreasing the dose. Then he became very technical.'

Jane did not improve even on the much higher dose of diamorphine to reduce her pain and of Valium to deal with her anxiety. She couldn't sleep; the drugs seemed only to induce a kind of stupor in her.

Dr. Murray came back and Victor waited outside again while he talked to Jane. Impatiently, Victor looked into the room through the little window in the door and saw that they had stopped talking. Jane was relaxing and Dr. Murray was sitting by her bed, holding her hand, watching her. Victor's own tension eased, and he felt an enormous sense of relief.

One of the night nurses sat with Jane while Dr. Murray spoke to Victor. It had been a long day for the doctor and he looked weary, but he took time to explain Jane's condition to her father.

The pain, he said, was everywhere, but he was now sure they could relieve it and he had made this clear to Jane. She wanted to know about pain in general, and he had explained that, too. Pain was not just a sensation, he told Victor. Aristotle, when he formulated his doctrine of the five senses – seeing, hearing, touching, taste, smell – had specifically excluded pain, which he described as the passion of the soul.

'I'm sure that would have appealed to Jane,' Victor told him. 'No other doctor has talked to her about Aristotle.'

Pain, Dr. Murray said, was an experience greater than a sensation, and it varied according to the mood and morale of the patient. They would have to work on that with Jane, no less than on the physical sources. Indeed, the physical sensations could be modified by the patient's emotional and psychological reactions to the pain. In Jane's case, her resistance to pain would have been lowered by her recent experiences. She hadn't been sleeping properly at night, so she was worn out. There were other discomforts, too, nausea, itching, anxiety, bad dreams, no bowel movement for several days, dry mouth, parched lips . . . All this, Dr. Murray said, could make the pain worse.

'We have to raise the patient's morale, and by treating these symptoms, we do just that, raise the morale and reduce the experience of pain. We moisten a dry mouth, clear out the bowels, give an injection against nausea – by correcting certain factors, we elevate the pain threshold. Depending on these actions, the same pain can be an agony or merely an ache.

'Look at it this way,' he went on. 'If a child gets hurt, it may be in agony until the mother caresses the hurt area, or offers an ice cream, a sweet or a kiss. These things can reduce the agony – real, genuine agony – to an ache. Haven't you seen this happen?'

'Yes, but a bruised knee is a momentary pain . . .'

'It's the same basic experience in a child and in an advanced cancer patient. Make sure that Jane has a good night's sleep, rest, sympathy and understanding from those around her and she'll . . .'

'But she had all the sympathy and understanding she needed at home.'

'I'm sure she did,' Dr. Murray replied soothingly, 'and she'll need it here, too, which is why it's so good that you're all going to be here. I'm certain your doctor gave her every drug he knew about, but he reached a point when it wasn't doing much good. You were just sitting there worrying, seeing she was getting worse – that's what you told me. And she was watching you, she knew what you were thinking, why you were worrying, and this increased her own anxiety. You thought that nothing could be done about it all, and she sensed it and believed it, even though you were telling her the opposite. But here, we can tell her, and show her, that as far as her pain's concerned she's getting better, that we're bringing it under control. She'll feel it happening, and believe us. Once her pain starts receding, she'll *expect* it to get better instead of worse. Her morale will improve. First we'll arrest it, then we'll start to roll it back.'

'But you haven't arrested it so far, have you?'

'Not yet, but she's dozed off and that's a good beginning. If we can give her a good night's sleep, then a comfortable rest during the day, so that she doesn't move around too much and the pain on movement is reduced, her mood will improve, her morale will be better, and she'll cope with the pain.'

When Dr. Murray had examined her, the pain was in both arms, in her neck and her back, in her abdomen. If he moved any of her limbs, any part of her body, she reacted with complaints that all movement was painful. This was what they had to overcome, and the drugs should begin to work now. She needed a lot of diamorphine, far more than the average patient, and he'd spoken to her quite frankly about the possible effects.

'I told her, as I'm telling you now, that she's bound to become confused for a time. She's been given new, powerful drugs. She's very ill. She's been moved from familiar to unfamiliar surroundings. She might wake in the night and become disoriented. That's one reason I'm glad you're going to be with her. If you speak to her and she recognises you, that will help a great deal, instead of her just lying there, wondering who she is, where she is, until a nurse comes – a nurse she might not know.'

He had warned Jane about it quite deliberately, and he was warning Victor now, so that they shouldn't be upset when it happened. 'It should take some of the fear away,' he said. 'If you have overwhelming pain, if you are demoralised with extreme anxiety, as Jane is, this could result in night-mares. If you're just starting on these new drugs, there is a considerable likelihood of these fears and anxieties coming out as drug-precipitated hallucinations. Then there might be misperceptions, and it is important to distinguish between all of these and to realise that they will ease after a few days. They will become less.'

'But surely she's not going to get better. She can only get worse. Doesn't that mean that the hallucinations will also get worse?'

'No. We're not trying to cure her,' the doctor stressed, 'but that doesn't mean she can only get worse. Our aim is to make her feel better, and I am confident that, with your coopera-tion, we should be able to achieve this, even as her illness deepens. Indeed, without our experience here, it might be assumed that as she becomes more ill she would hallucinate more frequently. But we've studied the process, and we know something of the causes and effects. We can tell you that after a few days the hallucinations are going to be reduced. I also told her this.' Dr. Murray wanted to give Jane something she could recognise as a success in the treatment in order to build up her confidence. This would help him too, he explained to Victor. 'Provided a doctor understands what's going on, he can cope. When a doctor feels powerless, his confidence goes. And when that happens, there is no hope of the patient's own confidence rising, and you go into an ever-increasing circle of depression.'

Victor was still worried. Would she become completely doped? His generation had little experience of drugs, and his questions reflected fear and mistrust.

Yes, the doctor conceded, they were increasing Jane's medication, but only so that they could cut down on it later. In an ordinary hospital, a doctor would normally prescribe painkilling drugs to be given to the patient every few hours, or 'as required'. If the prescription was for every two hours, then the patient had to wait, even if the pain had increased in the meantime. If it was 'as required', then the sufferer was dosed only when the pain had increased – by which time it was too late.

The hospice did it differently. 'You don't wait until the pain returns. You want to prevent this, to get on top and keep ahead of pain. You know from your patient's case history that the pain will come back. The idea is that you give the next dose *before* the effect of the previous one has worn off. So you establish the dose that'll do the trick, and you give it regularly. You anticipate pain, you don't wait for it to recur.'

As for addiction, Dr. Murray had made a study reviewing the case histories of five hundred patients to determine the effects of diamorphine. The results showed that the rate at which the dose increased became progressively less the longer the duration of the treatment. Addiction wasn't a problem, nor was excessive drowsiness.

In the majority of patients, Dr. Murray assured Victor, it was possible to achieve pain control while the patient was fully alert, and that, he explained, was what hospice treatment was all about. 'What patients want is to be free of pain, to be alert to live what life they have left, but in some situations it isn't possible to control pain completely, and the patient should then be warned, as I have warned Jane, that she may feel some distress when she moves. If a patient is told what's happening, and why, she will accept it and cope, and this will reduce a lot of the anxiety associated with chronic severe pain. Jane wanted the explanation; her questions showed that she understood it, I think she'll cope.'

Victor was more relaxed after his talk with Dr. Murray, and he found Jane was, too. She was exchanging a few words with Julia when he came in. Jane had been struck by the fact that Julia, the nursing officer in charge of the hospice, should have given up a night's rest to stand in for an absent nurse. She told Julia how impressed she was by the lack of hierarchical barriers.

'That's just the kind of remark I'd expect to hear from a social science student,' Julia said pleasantly, letting Jane know that she was familiar with her background.

But it was the wrong thing to say. Social science students had been in the van of student rebellion. Jane was inclined to see any such remark, when uttered by a middle-class square, as a challenge.

'Social science students are just as good as anyone else,' she exploded. 'What have you got against them? Why is everyone so foul?'

It was quite unreasonable, but perhaps it was her way of complaining about the pain. Julia was taken aback by the outburst she'd provoked and tried to explain she hadn't meant to offend, but Jane wouldn't listen. She sank into her pillow, an angry expression on her face. Her gratitude had turned to something like fury. Her eyes were saying to her father: 'Take these people away.'

'But Jane,' he protested, 'you know Julia didn't mean it that way.'

Was she going to alienate one member of the staff after the other? First Patricia, now Julia. Might the nurses come to shun her, or to treat her less kindly? Victor still thought of the hospice as a hospital, and followed Julia out of the room to apologise.

'We don't have many people here with overwhelming pain,' she said reassuringly. 'Jane has had so much she probably can't imagine it will go away. That's all she's thinking about. That was a sign of her anxiety. She hasn't settled in yet, she's not on our wavelength. I expected too much too soon.'

There obviously was no need to be concerned about antagonising the nurses, Julia was being almost apologetic herself in order to comfort him. Victor could afford to admit to her that Jane was sometimes difficult. 'She can take offence rather easily, particularly when she's ill. We used to tease her when she was a child and call her "Miss Umbrage".'

Julia smiled. 'We'll get her into a better frame of mind. It takes twenty-four to forty-eight hours to bring pain under control. When we've done that, Jane won't take umbrage.'

'Do you really think you can do it?'

'We'll certainly try. She mightn't always be free of pain but she'll know that we can help her. Then if the pain does reappear, it won't seem so bad to her because she'll know we should be able to make it go away again. There's a difference between a pain you know will go away, and one that you think won't.'

Julia realised that this night would be crucial. They had to break the cycle of pain and fear and make up for the time lost during the day when Jane's confidence in the promise of the hospice had been so undermined. She wanted to make sure she could give Jane as high a dose of diamorphine, as wide a selection of drugs, as might be necessary during the night. But a sister cannot give a patient whatever drugs she thinks are appropriate, even in a hospice. What she could do, and what Julia did, was to discuss with the doctor the likely course of events and anticipate what might happen: an increase in the intensity of pain, the appearance of a new source of pain, a bout of nausea. Julia mentioned to Dr. Murray the drugs she might require if Jane's condition changed, and found he had already prescribed them. That meant she wouldn't need to call him during the night. He had prescribed a wide range of doses, between 20 and 60 milligrams of diamorphine. The injections were to be given 'one to three hourly,' which meant that if Jane's pain eased, she need have no more than 20 milligrams every three hours; but if it went up, or showed no signs of abating, she could receive as much as 60 milligrams every hour – which is what Julia did in fact have to give her for several consecutive injections.

It was a bad night. Jane had dozed off at first, but she was soon wide awake. The pain seemed to ease slightly, then it returned with renewed force, racking her body so that she kept moving her upper limbs in anguish, which caused additional pain. Her lower limbs had become increasingly lifeless, as if paralysed. With each new wave of pain she opened her eyes wide, stared at Victor with mute reproof, and moved her hand slightly, very slightly, inside his. This was enough to transmit to him the current that was passing through her, to make him feel with her, to clench his own teeth in the hope that he could somehow help her.

Julia came by about every twenty minutes. Victor stretched out on his bed beside Jane's, holding her hand. The dose, which was 20 milligrams when Julia came on duty, was increased to 40, then to 60 at two o'clock in the morning, and again at three o'clock. Victor didn't sleep much during the night. Every time Jane stirred, he opened his eyes to watch, in the half-light, the expression of pain so often on her face. Earlier, the pain was intense, but localised. Now it was red-hot in her back but all-pervading, reaching down her trunk and into her hips, clawing at her stomach, pouring into her limbs. Every time Julia came in with another injection, Jane complained of pain.

At last she slept, uneasily, fitfully. She had been given enough diamorphine during that night, a doctor told Victor later, to kill an ordinary person. He was wrong. Jane was an ordinary person. But many general practitioners without specialised training in pain control are afraid of what they believe is the excessive use of a drug – until they have an opportunity to learn how beneficial it can be when administered by a doctor who knows what he is doing.

That night, they had given Jane enough diamorphine not to kill her but to break the cycle of pain and fear.

Victor would not know that until the next morning.

Chapter 10

The sound of the breakfast trolley woke Victor, who saw a face peering in through the window in the door. It was one of the kitchen maids checking if Jane was ready for breakfast. Jane was still sleeping and Victor heard the trolley move on. He was relieved she hadn't been disturbed. She needed the rest so badly. Even in her sleep, the pain lines on each side of her mouth, where in happier days there might have been a dimple, were deeply etched. Her face had set in an expression which conveyed the presence of pain through sharp creases, so unlike the natural wrinkles of old age.

As he watched, Jane stirred without opening her eyes. He covered her hand with his. Her hand moved slightly in reply. He said quietly, 'It's eight o'clock, Jane, and it's a beautiful morning. The sun's streaming down. Shall I draw the curtains?' He waited for her to answer.

'No.' Her voice was faint but distinct. 'The light will hurt my eyes. I want to keep them shut.'

'You can do that if I draw the curtains just a little.' He wanted her to face the new day, to stay in touch with reality.

'I don't want to open my eyes,' she said with sudden vehemence.

Another face peered in and it was Adela. He gestured for her to come in.

'How did you sleep, all right?' she asked cheerfully.

He was about to reply when Jane suddenly spoke up, still without opening her eyes: 'It's you, Adela, isn't it? I know your voice.'

Adela beamed. 'Aren't you clever! How did you manage it with your eyes shut?'

'It's your accent,' Jane murmured. 'Is it Greek?'

'No, but you're not far off. Would you like to try again, dear?'

But Jane was in no mood to play games. 'I don't want to think, I'm so tired.' Then she added more warmly: 'Could you stay with me? My father has to go now.'

That surprised Victor. He was ready to interrupt when Adela said quickly: 'I must say hello to the others – it won't take a jiffy – then I can stay with you for a while.'

She signalled to Victor to come out with her. She whispered to him, 'I think you could help Jane best now by leaving her alone for a bit.' She added: 'You've been with her all this time, and she wants a rest from you.'

He looked hurt. 'You need a rest from her too,' she said more gently. 'It's only natural.' Victor nodded stiffly and walked away.

When Adela returned to Jane's room, she soon learned what was worrying her. First Jane wanted to be sure Victor had gone, then she burst out: 'Oh, Adela, I'm so frightened! I can't open my eyes, my eyelids are so heavy. I can't see anything. I couldn't tell him. What is it? I can't see! I can't see!'

Adela touched her hand reassuringly. 'It's all right, dear. It's nothing to worry about, only the effect of all the drugs you've had to help your pain. That's why you feel so drowsy, so heavy, and so do your eyes. It'll pass away soon; just rest now as much as you can. If you feel like talking, talk – but don't worry about it.'

Adela's quiet confidence was catching, and as they chatted Jane seemed to grow stronger. The effect of the drugs receded, her eyelids no longer felt glued together. But the drowsiness made her feel strange.

'Am I drunk, Adela?'

'No, dear, you're as sober as I am. You were a little confused earlier, but I think you're fine now.'

'The pain's not as bad as it was, not now, but it'll come back, won't it? It always comes back worse than ever.' The creases in Jane's face deepened.

'It doesn't have to start up again,' Adela said. 'People sometimes come here in terrible pain and in a few days we get them better. Then they can go home and come back only if they need something special – or a change from their relatives!'

'People go home from here?' Now Jane opened her eyes wide, trying to see Adela's expression. 'You don't have to say things like that to me. I know where I am. This is a hospice, people come here to die. I'm not afraid of that . . . I don't think so . . . It's the pain I'm afraid of.'

'People do go home from here.' Adela said gently. 'I don't know if you will, you may prefer to stay. There's no parking meter by your bed. But your pain will ease, I'm sure of that. And if you do go home, there'll always be a bed kept ready for you here in case you need it.'

Adela began sponging Jane's face with a touch as gentle as a feather. She managed to slip her nightgown off and wash her body all over, but then decided the pain in her back was still too sharp to risk putting the nightgown on again.

'I know how we can make it easier,' she said. 'Let's put a pyjama top on.'

'That would be even worse,' Jane cried. 'My arms feel a bit better today, but I couldn't move them enough to get into sleeves. I just couldn't!'

'Of course not, dear. That's not what I meant,' Adela said quickly. 'We'll put it on back to front, so as not to hurt your back. You hardly need move your arms, we'll slip one arm into the sleeve in front of you, then the other . . .' She raised Jane's arm a little to see how she would react.

It was still painful, but not as bad as yesterday. 'I suppose I can do it if I have to,' Jane said, 'but what's the point of wearing pyjamas or a nightgown? I like sleeping with nothing on, that's how I sleep at home. I'd have liked to sleep naked at the hospital, too, but I never dared ask.' She looked up at Adela. 'Do you think they'd mind very much if I stayed like this? After all, there's the sheet over me. Could you ask – maybe the sister in charge?'

Adela didn't need to ask anyone's permission. 'Of course you needn't wear your nightie,' she said. 'All that matters is that you should feel comfortable.'

'I know some people would be shocked by the sight of a

naked body, but we're not like that in my family. I feel more natural like this, so why pretend?'

'You don't have to pretend here, Jane.'

Jane's eyes were wide open now. She was more ready to talk.

'Do I still have to guess where you come from?' she asked.

'No, I'm quite willing to tell you if you don't want to work it out for yourself.'

Adela's jet-black hair was one clue. Jane still couldn't see her features very clearly. There was something Semitic about her appearance, but she was sure Adela wasn't Jewish. She felt she had enough Jewish blood herself to tell instinctively whether someone else was a Jew.

'I thought you might be Greek because your accent seemed familiar. I was teaching in Greece a few months ago. Have I got the right part of the world?'

'You're not too far off.'

'The Mediterranean?'

'Warm. Try again.'

'The Middle East, then.'

'That's very warm.'

'You're an Arab?'

Adela smiled warmly. 'You see, you got it by yourself, Jane. Yes, I come from Syria. Did you teach geography?'

'No, but I've travelled quite a bit. I went on a trip round the world with Dad when I was fifteen, and that took in the Middle East.'

'Did you go to Syria?'

'No, but we stopped off in Israel. How do you feel about Israel?' Jane didn't want to lose her new friend. She'd known Arabs who became hostile even at the mention of Israel.

'I've been back to Syria several times since the war,' Adela answered carefully. 'Did you know that there are Jews there, and they get on quite well with the Syrians? It's the politicians who make the trouble, not ordinary people.'

Jane felt she could talk more freely. 'I liked Israel a lot. I went back to work on a kibbutz the following summer. There's something about kibbutz life that makes you want to come back – I even thought of living there for good. Then one day I saw some Arabs being searched by the police. They took a man away. He was scared, he didn't want to go with them. He argued, but it was no good. They started pushing him towards the police car, and he fell. It was a field road. He fell into the dust.'

Adela and Jane talked more that morning, about Jews and Arabs, about each other's families, about the lives they had led. Soon they knew each other quite well. She had made a new friend, Jane told Rosemary happily on her return a little later.

It had seemed a long night to Rosemary. She looked anxiously to see if there were any changes. The previous afternoon, Jane hadn't been able to move her head on the pillow; now she could turn slowly towards her mother. But her eyes were large and sluggish, and her face puffy from the drugs. Her lips moved slowly and her voice was soft: 'Am I dying, Mum?'

'Not just yet, darling,' Rosemary replied calmly. 'It won't be much longer, though. And we'll stay with you. It will be soon.' Rosemary wished she could be more specific and tell her exactly when. She knew Jane wanted to get it over with before the decay of her body overtook her mind.

'I hope it isn't long,' Jane murmured. 'I don't want it to be long.'

'We know we have to lose you – what's important is that you should be as comfortable as you can until it happens. They are determined to make it as easy as possible for you here.'

'I feel so sleepy . . .' Her voice was hazy.

'We don't have to talk. Just rest. I'll be here if you wake up and need anything.' Once more Rosemary felt torn by her conflicting emotions – wishing that death would come quickly, yet still hoping for one of those miraculous reversals. When Jane was dead, there would be no hope left.

Rosemary looked around the room. Yesterday had been too full of anguish for casual inspections. It was a warm place. Yesterday it had been a sick room; now it was a bedroom, a place of retreat overlooking a garden. Jane couldn't see as far as the bird table outside and the flowers planted in tubs on a terrace, nor to the trees bordering the golf course. But the door to the terrace was open, and she could experience the sounds and smells of June. Perhaps soon she would feel well enough to have her bed pushed through the wide door into the open air, so that she could watch the birds and enjoy the flowers.

There was no sinister-looking chart clipped to the bed. Nobody had produced a plastic identification bracelet with the instruction that it must be worn at all times. Jane had hated the bracelets, always tearing them off as soon as she was out of the hospital door. But here in the hospice she was already well known to the entire staff.

She stirred and opened her eyes. 'Mum, do they know how ill I am?' she asked anxiously. 'Do they know I'm going to die?'

Rosemary stroked the hand she held. 'Yes, they know. They talk to us about it and about what they're doing to help you. Everyone is very kind.'

'And where do we go when we have to leave?' It was another reminder of her completely helpless state, of the total lack of control over either her body or her future, and of the insecurity she had come to feel in the months of wandering from hospital to hospital.

'We don't have to leave here.' Rosemary spoke slowly, stressing the words. 'We can stay as long as we want. When they get your pain under control, we can take you home, but only if that's what you want. It'll be up to you to decide.' Perhaps even the thought of another journey would be too much for Jane. 'We can stay here as long as you wish,' she repeated.

Jane seemed satisfied, and sank slowly back into sleep. The room was quiet and peaceful until suddenly there came the sound of violent ꞏetching from the bedroom next door. It sounded like an old man in considerable distress. Jane winced, but said nothing. Footsteps hurried past, then came the voices of Dr. Murray and one of the nurses. It was obviously an emergency. Dr. Murray was due to visit Jane, but we heard him talk on and on next door. It was one time when Jane wasn't irritated to be kept waiting.

He arrived at last in his shirt sleeves, without the usual white coat. 'May I come in?' Rosemary left him alone with Jane.

Half asleep, she looked vacantly at him, but as he sat

down, she smiled. He allowed time for her to adjust to his presence before he spoke.

'You may not remember I came to see you last night, you were in such pain. My name is David Murray.' He enunciated slowly, giving her a chance to remember.

'I know,' Jane said quite clearly. 'We met yesterday.'

'How are things today?' he asked, as he took her pulse. He continued to hold her wrist lightly, gently, almost as if it were a substitute for shaking hands.

'The pain isn't as bad as it was,' Jane confirmed.

She felt like a human being again, with distinct thoughts and varied sensations of her own. The overwhelming sense of pain that had so recently blotted out her personality had subsided. But she needed to restore her sense of self. Dr. Murray knew that Jane's hospital experience had given her a fear of regimentation, and he wanted to make it clear that she didn't have to be anxious about that at the hospice. He spoke about getting to know her as an individual. Everyone's reactions were so different, he said. 'We want to find out what suits you, Jane. Is there anything you need?'

'I wish I had my tape recorder here.'

'That's easy,' he assured her. 'There's a small portable recorder in the lounge for the patients. What type of music do you like?'

'These days I only seem to enjoy classical music – quiet things.'

'I think we have some tapes for you.' They talked about the composers they both liked. If Jane could discuss music, she must be feeling much better than the day before. She needed strength for the future. He had to help her handle whatever might happen next. He usually tried to give his patients full awareness of what was going on by explaining anything that puzzled them. He wanted the patient to know that this doctor understood what was happening, understood what he was talking about, and realise: 'Now I don't have to worry any more.'

Jane still had some problems apart from the pain – hallucinations and drowsiness. Dr. Murray talked to her about them.

He explained that the drowsiness was caused by the

injections, which were designed to ease her pain. But the pain was already lessening, and he was thinking of changing the combination of drugs. Her body had to have time to adjust. They were still experimenting to see what suited her best. Nor was the drowsiness necessarily a bad sign. Her body required rest after all it had been through.

'I don't find the hallucinations restful,' Jane told him.

'I did warn you about them.'

'You said they'd stop after a time. But they frighten me.'

'They're caused by the drugs I'm giving you, and should ease off after a while. If not, there are one or two things I can try to do about it. Just so long as we know they are hallucinations . . .'

'What else could they be?'

'This may be too fine a distinction for you, Jane, but hallucinations are one thing and misperceptions are another. You've been having hallucinations, and that's why I know we can put things right. We've studied the field quite thoroughly.'

He watched her carefully. Could she take it all in?

'What is a hallucination, then?' she asked.

'I can give you the scientific definition, if you really want it.'

'Please.'

'A hallucination is an auditory, visual, or olfactory experience which arises independently of an external stimulus.'

Jane smiled as if she had heard enough.

'How long will it be before I die?' She needed to know how much time was left for all that remained to be done. But he in turn had to be sure that she was really ready for the truth.

'Before you came here, Dr. Sullivan told you it would probably be weeks rather than months?'

'Yes, but that's not really saying much, is it? It's been going on for weeks already. I don't want it to last too long.'

'I don't think you have much further to go, Jane,' David Murray said softly. No other doctor had spoken to her with such a matter-of-fact acceptance of death. 'Quite how long it will be, I just don't know – not at the moment. Let's control the pain first, and then see how you are. Ask me again in a few days, I may be able to give you a better idea.'

'But I am going to die now, aren't I?' Jane seemed to be seeking reassurance. 'In the hospital, they wouldn't tell me. Everyone said something different, it didn't make sense.'

'Yes, Jane, you are going to die. But we'll be here to help you through it. Nobody will lie to you here. You can ask anything you want to know and we'll answer your questions. If we don't know the answer, we'll try to find out. We're all well trained, and we've had a good deal of experience.'

She moved her hand slightly toward him – as far as she could – and he held it. 'Everyone has been so good,' she murmured, 'but you have helped me most, Dr. . . .' she waited for him to repeat his name.

'Murray.'

He made her feel secure. She could talk easily, freely, to him about what was happening to her, about life – and death. He was a doctor she could fully trust, at last. She felt very close to him.

'I can't keep calling you Dr. Murray,' she said.

'Call me David. Everyone else does.'

Victor and Rosemary were also favourably impressed with Dr. Murray. We realised he was going to help Jane through the process of dying, not try to cure her, as others had promised. There had been so many doctors. At times Jane had seemed like the baton in a relay race, passed from one hand to another as each stage of her illness ended and a new phase began. Now at the very end she had once again found a man she could trust, a fitting successor to our family physician, Dr. Sullivan. And he reflected the quality of the people who worked with him. In the hospice, doctors, nurses and auxiliary helpers formed a close team. The nurses had come to the hospice from different backgrounds, with varying individual experiences, and they sometimes differed on how a patient should be handled. The discussion between Pat and Julia about drugs for Jane was an example of that. But they combined their experiences and thrashed out their differences in a way that served to strengthen their relationship with the patients and with each other.

Jane was moved frequently in the bed so that her joints

wouldn't stiffen and cause her more pain. She seemed more relaxed, and was soon lying on her side – a major achievement. Always before she had refused to change her position, afraid that any move might increase her suffering. But Adela explained that occasional changes in the way she was lying would protect her from bedsores. Lying on her right side, she was no longer a passive, helpless patient staring into space. She had the confidence to vary her position. She could also see a little better and was able to take more part in what was happening in her room.

Adela's attempts to get Jane to eat were typical of her whole approach. 'When my children had no appetite we used to play games together,' she said, shaping the food with a spoon. 'What do you think that is meant to be?' She held up a moulded lump of potato.

'I really can't be sure.' Jane giggled slightly. 'It might be . . . a duck?'

'It is a duck,' Adela said firmly. 'One, two, three, and it's in your mouth!'

Jane swallowed it obediently.

They played a game that went easily from the make-believe situation of a mother feeding her child to the reality of one adult helping the other. Jane couldn't have played with her own mother and pretended to be a child again, but she could do it with a comparative stranger like Adela. They had become so close that when Adela went off duty for two days, we feared Jane would be upset. Adela promised to try to call in, and Jane seemed content.

That evening she started to go to sleep, then suddenly her eyes opened wide, focusing sharply on Rosemary. 'Have you just lost half your face? There's a gap below your nose.'

Rosemary laughed uneasily and put her hand to her face. 'No, you're wrong. I can feel it's all there. It must be another hallucination, Jane.'

Sometimes the hallucinations worried her, but Dr. Murray's explanations helped her to come to terms with them. 'David said they should ease off after a while,' she assured us.

Victor was sitting with her when, with a wicked smile, she informed him that his face was 'quite funny.' His ear was where his nose should be, his eye was in his chin, and there was a gaping hole in his forehead through which, she said, she could see the sky. When he looked distressed, she consoled him. 'It's rather like a good Picasso,' she said. The next time this happened, she said she could only see half of his face, inordinately elongated. 'Very interesting,' she chuckled. What, he asked, another Picasso? No, she answered thoughtfully, rather like a Modigliani.

After seeing her again, David Murray was not worried by these hallucinations. He told us: 'She's much more alert now. I hear she's chatting with Adela quite a lot. It's good to see them developing a personal relationship. The drugs help, but they can't do everything.'

'We wouldn't want to take Adela away from the other patients,' Rosemary said tentatively, 'but it would be good if she could spend as much time as possible with Jane.'

'I think it could be arranged. Certain patients take more to particular nurses and' – he looked up with a smile – 'less to others.' Had he heard about Patricia? 'These things usually work themselves out.'

'Now that Adela's off duty for two days,' Victor asked, 'will Jane maintain her improvement?'

'Yes, we've got things under control. With the pain receding, and Jane more aware of her surroundings, she'll be getting to know the other nurses.'

'But the pain receded only when you increased the dose of diamorphine,' Victor said. 'How long can you go on stepping it up?'

'I think she's stabilised,' David answered. 'Now that I know where the pain is worst and where it comes from – her arms, for instance – there are other actions we can take. Like a nerve block.'

'We promised her no more operations,' Rosemary exclaimed. 'I thought you agreed with us.'

'I do. We might very rarely operate for palliative purposes, to ease the pain, but a nerve block isn't an operation.'

'Does it matter what you call it?' Victor was not reassured. 'Once you cut the nerve, you can't tie it up again, can you? She'd never have any feeling again in that area, neither pain nor anything else.'

'We're not going to cut anything, and it's not irreversible. Let me try to explain.'

But we didn't want to hear any more. We had been talked into so many things we didn't really want at the hospital, so many treatments. 'We don't want to go through all that again,' Victor said petulantly.

'I won't try to talk you into anything you don't want, I assure you,' Dr. Murray went on, with his usual deliberation. 'I'm not even sure myself that this is something we should do. I was merely thinking aloud. I thought you'd like to know what the possibilities are.'

'If it will control her pain, perhaps we ought to think about it,' Victor said, rather shamefaced. 'It's been a long day, we're a bit on edge. But much better than yesterday, thanks to you.'

'Don't thank me yet.' He looked at them both. 'But I think we're making progress.'

It was Rosemary's turn to stay the night with Jane. They had asked us whether we would rather take turns at going home to rest or both stay at the hospice. We didn't want to leave. Home was where Jane was. So they gave us a room with two beds. Victor found that there was another visitor's bedroom next to it, unoccupied, and soon he moved in his own papers and files. He still had a newspaper column to write. When Jane had learned, at Dairy Cottage, that she might not have much time left, Victor told her he would give up writing his column for the duration of the illness so that he could devote himself completely to her. Jane's reply was to cry out in mock horror, 'Help!' She made him promise that he would keep up the column whatever happened. She did not, she said, want him to devote himself completely to her or there might be trouble. Now, at the hospice, the staff told Victor he could use the second room as a study so long as it was not needed for other relatives. He had not missed a single column throughout her illness, and it was important to him, for Jane's sake, that he should not miss one now. As Rosemary settled down for the night in Jane's room, Victor went to work in his new study.

Nora, a young night nurse, came to give Jane her midnight injection. She tried not to wake her too suddenly.

'Just a little jab now, Jane.'

Jane stirred and peered into the half-light. 'Is my mother still here?' she murmured. 'I'd like someone to talk to.'

'I think she's asleep,' Nora said gently. She was about Jane's age and identified strongly with her. 'Do you want me to stay a bit? I've got plenty of time.'

It didn't take Nora long to put Jane at her ease. 'It's not that I'm afraid of dying,' Jane confided. 'I'm scared the pain will get bad again and that I'll go to pieces.'

'We won't let that happen,' Nora said firmly. 'We'll help you as long as you need us.'

'It's my father who needs help,' Jane said.

'In what way?'

'He had a bad time in the war. I don't think he's ever got over it.'

'Got over what?'

'I don't really know. He won't talk about it.'

'Perhaps he will now that your pain's more under control.'

Nora had seen many families come together in the hospice. Talk was sometimes more truthful when death was close. It was her hope that Jane could help her father.

Chapter 11

In the night Rosemary awoke suddenly to find Jane's eyes wide open with a look of fear.

'Mum. Are you there?'

Rosemary bent over so that Jane could see her and feel her touch.

'Yes, I'm right here.'

'Mum, I'm absolutely terrified. Where are we? What is this place?'

Rosemary kissed her to try to drive away the nightmare. 'Jane, it's quite all right. We're in the hospice near Oxford and everyone is wonderful. They've been working to reduce your pain, and you're much better.'

'It's another hospital?'

'No, it's completely different. When you wake up properly, you'll remember how much you like it here.'

'We're still in England?' Her eyes remained wide open and frightened.

'Yes. Dad's asleep just down the corridor, and Richard and Arloc will be with you tomorrow morning.'

She wasn't convinced. 'I still don't get it. Can we go over it again?'

Rosemary repeated her reassurances, but Jane's eyes remained troubled.

'I'll ask Nora to fetch Dad. If you see him, it might help.'

A few minutes later Victor padded in on bare feet. Rosemary explained Jane's confusion while he bent over her, touching her. They switched the brighter lights on. Jane looked around suspiciously.

'But this isn't the same room I was in yesterday.'

'Yes, it is. You haven't been moved, and they won't move you.'

'No, Dad. It isn't the same.' Her eyes passed vaguely over the room. 'The furniture is different.' Her voice was firmer, surer. She was fully awake but still deeply suspicious.

'That's just because we moved everything round when you were asleep to make room for a cot for me.' Rosemary touched each piece of furniture. 'See, this cupboard was over here by your bed with a chair beside it. Now the chair is in the passage. There was another chair here, the other side of the bed, that's out in the passage, too.'

'The window looks different. It isn't in the same place.'

'That's only because the curtains are across the window. Look, I'll pull them back. There are stars in the sky.'

Jane still wasn't convinced. 'Are we in England now?' she asked again.

'Yes,' Victor repeated, 'in a hospice, near Oxford.'

Rosemary had an idea. 'Tomorrow, when we rearrange the furniture for the night, we'll do it before you go to sleep, Jane, so that you can watch us. That'll help you to remember.'

Slowly she began to relax.

Victor had had a good sleep in the visitors' room. He suggested he should stay with Jane now, while Rosemary took the more comfortable bed. But he had no sooner settled down in the cot than he heard Jane call out. 'Look, Dad, look.' She pointed to the foot of the bed. 'Make it go away!'

'What is it Jane?'

'There's the nasty little brute again.' She described to him the ratlike brown animal she could see scurrying across the bed. 'It's giving me the horrors!'

'All right, Jane, let's make it go away together. If you can see the little brown animal, then you must know he's in a field, not on your bed. Can you see the field?'

'Ye-es,' Jane said doubtfully.

'A beautiful green field with the grass bending in the wind,' he continued evenly, almost hypnotically. 'Tall, green grass. Wavelike. With beautiful wild flowers – red poppies, very red.'

'Yes,' she confirmed, this time with more assurance. The little brown animal had gone. 'Red poppies,' she repeated easily.

'The field is on a slope, the wind is blowing uphill, the sun is shining and it's a hot summer day – not a cloud in the sky. A blue, blue sky. . . .'

'No,' Jane interrupted him suddenly, almost angrily. 'There's no hill. There's a field, but no hill.'

'Oh?'

'It's very flat. There's a small stream, then there's the field. And a cottage with a thatched roof.' She was describing the house where we lived when we were first married.

'There's a garden by the stream. Yes, lots of flowers, red poppies.'

'Go on, Jane.' He began to feel uneasy. The picture was accurate, but . . . Then he knew in a flash, with a sense of shock, what was wrong. She was describing something she couldn't have known. Jane had never lived in that house, we had moved from there before she was born.

'But, Jane . . .'

'Richard is in the garden, and I'm angry. Richard is there, and you and Mum are there. But I'm not there. I'm very angry.'

Victor didn't know what to say. Dr. Murray had warned him about nightmares and hallucinations, not visions.

'But, Jane, that was before you were born,' he said finally.

'That's why I'm so angry. Richard was there, and you and Mum, but not me.'

No, it wasn't a vision, he thought, it was like something out of Freud. She'd always been a little jealous of Richard. So many things that were difficult for her seemed to be easy for him. Jane's old feelings must be rising to the surface again. But how could she know what the place looked like if she hadn't been there? His sense of unease deepened. He managed to change the subject to her own childhood, to some of the happy times she'd had. Then, suddenly, the explanation came to him.

'Jane, that cottage, the garden, the stream . . . It wasn't before you were born. We had moved out of there, and then – you were about four or five – we went back to see the cottage. We were together that day, you and Richard, all of us. That's what you remembered.'

But she was no longer interested. The anger had subsided. They went on reminiscing easily like two old friends. Jane didn't want to go back to sleep, she wanted to talk. When he asked about the pain, she dismissed the question with a very slight movement of her hand – a better answer than any other she could have given, because it showed how the pain in her arm had subsided. He was amazed at the improvement.

If he hadn't known how ill she was, how deeply the cancer had eaten into her, he would have thought she was beginning to heal. But, he asked Dr. Murray later, would she be as ready to die now that she appeared to be getting better? He wondered if she would begin to hope for a cure. Then all the good the hospice was doing her would be cancelled out.

And when Dr. Murray next saw Jane, he found the questions she was putting to him had changed. She wasn't asking about the pain, she wanted to know more about the disease. What was the cancer doing to her body, was it spreading? The present had completely preoccupied her when the pain was so intense. Now she was inquiring about the future. She didn't ask, 'Am I going to get better?' in so many words, yet Dr. Murray thought that perhaps the idea lay behind her questions. He told her of the tumour in her stomach, of the cancer in her bones, and explained what he was doing to control the distress this had caused her. The real answer to her question was, 'No, you're not going to get better,' but he did not put it so bluntly. The previous day he had marvelled at the equanimity with which she viewed the prospect of death. He had not often met such acceptance in someone so young. Yet it was just because of her youth that her attitude might alter. He could see now why Jane's shift of mood worried her father, and he decided he had to deal directly with Victor. He gave him as much time and attention as if he were a patient.

David Murray told Victor how it happened from time to time that dying patients changed their minds and abandoned their acceptance. 'Some come here in great pain, though not often in such agony as Jane, but we usually get it under control. Then, when the pain's relieved, they think they're getting better. They can't understand why they're still weak. There can be a simple equation in a patient's mind: Pain means I'm dying. No pain means I should be getting better.'

'Is Jane thinking this?'

'If she isn't, then she may at least be wondering about it. The relief of physical distress does cause a resurgence of determination, a reassertion of the will to live. In Jane's case, because she's so young, we have to reckon with the survival instinct. Even if she's intellectually prepared to die, even if she expects it and wants to get it over with, she may not be able to suppress the instinct to survive. It's a powerful force. There must be a lot of it left in her young body, and it could speak to her more loudly, more compellingly, than her intellect.'

'Then we must bring her back to reality,' Victor said firmly. 'We must tell her she *is* dying. Shall I do it, or would it be better if you did?'

'No, we needn't force the issue. You don't confront a patient with such information when she's not ready. She's already shown that she can accept death. This is something temporary – a change between yesterday and today that might be reversed again between today and tomorrow. Or even within an hour or two.'

When Victor returned to Jane's room and asked how she was feeling, she replied simply: 'Happy.'

Happy? What a word to use in the circumstances. And yet she had used it repeatedly, at Dairy Cottage when she was out of pain, and at the hospice once the pain was brought under control. She had used the word to describe her own state of mind, and urged Victor to share this with her. He pretended that he did – of course, he would do anything to make her happy. If she was happy, then so was he, or so he said, for the word meant nothing to him.

He couldn't fool her. Jane told him, 'Dad, you're just saying it. That's no good. There's only one way I know how to make you accept it – by a dialectical discussion.'

He had never before talked to her frankly about his own attitude to death, not in all those months when we thought of little else except her dying.

Once Dr. Sullivan had told her the truth, Jane began to turn the tables on her father. She was trying to tell him, first at Dairy Cottage and now at the hospice when the lines of communication were reopened between them, that he was hiding something.

'You must have faced death so many times, Dad,' she began carefully as he sat by her bed. 'You should be able to take this thing that's happening more easily than the rest of us.'

Victor guessed what she was leading up to and gave her a studied, factual answer. 'Yes, I suppose the first time was when I was about sixteen on the Russian–German front, after I got away from Siberia. I'm sure I've told you about it.'

'No, Dad, you haven't,' Jane said, watching him. 'You don't talk much about that time. I wish you would. What did happen?'

Should he tell her the full story? He had given her snatches of it over the years – his childhood in Poland, his wanderings during the war, the loss of his family, his escape from Russia – but always leaving out some important details. Now she had asked a specific question and he had to answer it.

'It was the summer the Germans attacked Russia, and by then I was right in the middle of it. I was on my own, the rest of my family had been swallowed up by the war.' He fell silent again.

'You were at the front?' she asked quietly.

'We were just behind the front, on the Russian side, mostly women, old people and youngsters like myself. We were driven like cattle, usually on foot, from one place to another, to dig anti-tank trenches which were supposed to stop the advancing Germans. But this time they loaded us into these carts because they were in a hurry to build a huge network of earth defences. We had driven past an army unit that seemed to be re-forming for the front, when suddenly all the soldiers dropped what they were doing and ran to take cover wherever they could. In less than a minute everything was still except for the horses prancing about and neighing. Then we could hear it . . . the drone of an airplane, not the powerful roar of the jet that your generation is used to, more like the sound of a motorcycle combined with the buzzing of a bumblebee, and perhaps overlaid by a lawnmower motor.'

'It's hard to imagine,' she prompted him. 'I'd like to know how it felt – to hear the sound of a plane about to bomb you.'

'Our cart and the tractor pulling it were the only things that kept going. We'd already moved well past the soldiers, but our driver must have decided to get even further away from them before the planes began bombing the troops. So the cart shook more than ever, but we didn't mind. We were looking up into the sky – at least I was, but I couldn't see anything. And then, in the distance, where the troops had been, I saw showers of earth being thrown up into the air, mixed with the debris of carts, trucks, men, horses – and only then came the explosions, punctuated with bursts of machine-gun fire which got closer and closer.

'We could see bullets kicking up the dust on the road a long way behind us. The driver took one look, cut the engine, and was off the tractor and into the ditch by the roadside almost before any of us had managed to get out of the cart. All the others followed him, but I thought I could do better. The ditch led to a culvert just a little way along the road, and I figured I was small enough to get right inside it. I stuck my head into the opening, but the rest of me was too big, and I was still struggling to push my way in when I heard more bombs, much louder, and at the same time I felt as if I was being beaten by powerful fists. Stones and clods of earth struck all over my body, but my head was safe. It lasted only a moment. I could hear cries and moaning. The plane had gone. I pulled my head out of the culvert and looked around. There wasn't much left of the tractor driver and one or two others. I was weak with fear, with a kind of delayed panic.' Victor stopped abruptly. It was years since he had thought about that day.

'I know,' Jane said after a pause. 'I think I know the feeling. It used to come to me in the hospital. It was the operations. I could take that. But after the operations, it would get to me. I used to think, "Am I ever going to escape from this?" And I'd be scared, panicky, and feel weak. I *was* weak, I wasn't eating very much.'

'You're not eating much these days, either. But you're not scared. At least, you don't seem to be.' He looked at her. 'Are you?'

'No, Dad,' she said. 'I'm not scared now and I hope I can stay unscared – if you help me. You helped me so much, at Dairy Cottage, when they first told me what was happening, and you just sat there and talked and talked to me.'

He touched her hand. 'Jane, you were ready for it. You'd lived with it for months and you needed no help from me. I was talking to help myself more than you.'

Victor felt unsure how to continue, sensing that something was still missing from their conversation. He had deliberately avoided talking of his own feelings about dying in his recollection of the bombing incident. Was that what Jane had wanted to hear?

She might have been reading his thoughts. 'But why were you at the front at sixteen?'

'What you have to understand, Jane, is that I had lost everybody, everything. When the war started and the Germans invaded Poland from the west and the Russians from the east, it wasn't just a war of soldiers. Everybody was on the move, whole populations were being shifted from place to place, or what remained of the populations after the troops had done their work. That's how I found myself in Siberia. But I escaped. I wanted to get back to a place where I belonged, where I could recognise the people, the buildings, the mountains in the distance. I was trying to get home to Poland, even though I knew that by now the Germans had driven most of the Jews off to concentration camps and imposed a regime of terror on the country. All this meant nothing to me compared with my urge to get back home, to find my roots again. I wasn't considering the danger. I suppose I even thought it exciting in a way – I'd join the partisans, be a hero. It was unrealistic, I suppose, but it was what I wanted, what I needed.'

Jane thought for a while. 'So you weren't running away from something, you were running *to* something?'

'It must have been six of one, half a dozen of the other. It wasn't just my own family I had lost. When the Russians put me in the prison camp, the people who had befriended me were finished off either by the Siberian winter, or the starvation diet, or the heavy labour or disease. And then, when I was let out of the prison camp – they said there had been a mistake, I was too young – there was the typhus epidemic. People were dropping dead like flies. That's when I decided I'd had enough.'

'To have had death all around you like that, when you were sixteen, must make you think,' she prompted him again.

'It certainly makes you run,' Victor replied. 'First I was running towards the front to get across it and make it back home, but that bombing raid changed my mind. I turned away from the Germans and went back into the interior of Russia.'

'Was that when you met Ilya Ehrenburg?'

'Yes. I made my way from the front all the way to the Volga, to Kuibyshev, which was where the whole Soviet government had retreated because the Germans were advancing on Moscow. And Ehrenburg had retreated with them, because he was one of the top Soviet writers, part of the government élite.'

'You never told me much about that. I only knew the part that was published in the history of the *Guardian*. At the school where I was teaching, one of the other teachers who had read the book wanted me to give her all the gory details. It was quite embarrassing. I couldn't tell her that my father never talked about the past to us, that he had some kind of guilty secret.' She smiled. 'Did you have one?'

'You know the story, you've heard it all before.'

'Only in bits and pieces. I'd like to hear it properly.'

He still hoped to escape her questioning, but she wouldn't let him. She had once told Victor that the Ehrenburg story might contain a key to something he was trying to hide. He had brushed her off then. He couldn't do it now. 'You really want to hear it all again?'

'You know I do, Dad – how, when, why, everything.'

He took a deep breath. 'In the winter of 1941–42, by the time I got to Kuibyshev, the town was full of evacuees, refugees, and troops, with thousands of people seeking shelter and hundreds huddling every night on the concrete floors of the main railway station, especially those whose status was somewhat dubious, like mine. If they'd found out that I had escaped from Siberia, I'd have been for it. I'd managed to get some false identity documents, and I was living from day to day, hand to mouth, as best I could, but even then I kept up my interest in what was going on. I read the papers which were pasted every day on the wall outside the station, and sometimes I managed to find a magazine. That's how I came across a piece by Ehrenburg one day, with a Kuibyshev dateline, so I knew he was there, and straight away I decided I would try to meet him.'

'But why him?'

'Because he'd been my hero for years – well, since about twelve or thirteen, I suppose, when I read his novel *Julio Jurenito*.'

'So *that's* why you tried to get me to read it. I wish you'd told me. If I'd known, I might have got beyond the first few pages.'

'That was during your anarchist period, Jane, and I knew better than to try to persuade you to do anything. I just left the book lying around hoping you'd recognise Julio Jurenito as a fellow anarchist and get as much out of it as I did during my anarchist period.'

'You didn't guess I'd see what you were up to?' Now she was smiling. 'You always did think I wasn't as clever as Richard.'

He ignored that. He wasn't about to discuss sibling rivalries at this point.

'Yes, Jane, you were a late developer.' He echoed her bantering tone. 'I must have been only about twelve when I became an anarchist. I don't think you got to it until your middle teens, by which age I was well beyond that phase. But I remembered the impression *Julio Jurenito* had made on me, like opening the door into a new world. I felt Ehrenburg was a kindred soul, somebody who'd understand my predicament, help me, maybe even get me some better place to sleep than the railway station. So I tracked him down and went to see him.'

'Just like that?'

'Yes, just like that, in rags, dirty, very much the street urchin in a great big army overcoat, the bottom cut off with a knife to stop it trailing on the ground. The edges were ragged because I had no scissors. For boots I cut up some car tyres, bound them together with string and rags, and stuffed the inside with bits of felt.'

Jane looked at him incredulously. 'That was your own invention?'

'No, it was a fairly common type of footwear then for down-and-outs. I'd got his address from the city address bureau, probably the only by-product of the police state that helped the citizen. You just went in, filled out a form with the name of the person whose address you wanted, and they gave it to you.'

'And you were allowed in to see him like that, rags and all?'

'He was out the first time I called, so I went back in the evening, said I was an admirer of his books, and he came to the door to see me. He asked me where I was from, and I said I was a refugee from German-occupied territory, all on my own. He wanted to know my age. I suppose he took pity on me, because he invited me in. My heart was beating so fast, I can still remember it. He was at the height of his fame – his books, his articles were everywhere. He was the great German-baiter, the man whose writings kept up Russian spirits at the time when they were suffering the most disastrous defeats of the war, and here was I being received by him, in the most luxurious apartment I'd ever seen.'

'So he wasn't an anarchist any more?'

'He asked me what books of his I'd read, and I blurted out, "*Julio Jurenito*." He went silent, quite rigid, for a moment, as if I'd said the worst thing possible, which of course I had. He wrote that book soon after the Revolution, long before Stalin had finished off all the anarchists, and it wasn't something he wanted to be reminded about. It must have been purged from all the libraries and burned by then. He probably didn't even have a copy of his own. In a way, that book stood for everything that Stalin had suppressed.'

'So you started off badly with him?'

'No, quite the contrary. Politically, it was the wrong thing to say; but personally, after that moment's silence, he warmed to me as if I was his long-lost son. It was obviously a book he cared for a great deal, more than the political hackwork he'd been doing in recent years. He'd put a lot of himself into that book, but probably no one had dared to mention it to him in years. It would have been dangerous if anyone had overheard him talking about it.'

He went on to explain how Ehrenburg got him some clean clothes, a place to live in, and a job as apprentice at the railway engineering works. They met once or twice a week. Victor told him the story of his life, carefully censored, though, because he had learned to distrust even his best friends. He even mentioned his secret ambition to be a writer, not just any writer, but one as influential as Ehrenburg. His benefactor smiled tolerantly, encouraged him to talk, told him something of his own life and struggles – not too much, though, because he wasn't taking any chances either. But before long the confidence, the intimacy which grew between them, made it possible for Ehrenburg to broach a subject more dangerous than any they had discussed so far.

'If you really want to be a writer,' he said, 'then you should be making some decisions now. You're Polish, you were born there, you went to school there, that's the culture you've absorbed. To be a Soviet writer, you'd have to start all over again, and you'd find it difficult. For you, this is a strange, foreign country . . .'

What Ehrenburg was trying to convey was that Victor should get out of the Soviet Union – and in time he told him how it could be done. The Poles who had been taken prisoner and deported to Russia at the beginning of the war, at the time of the Stalin–Hitler alliance, were now being released from the camps to join a new Polish army, which would fight at the Russians' side against their common German enemy. A small Polish air force unit was also being sent to England, so that its men could replenish the Polish squadrons which had lost so many of their pilots during the Battle of Britain. Victor must join this air force unit; but it wouldn't be easy. He should present himself at the recruiting station, say that he wanted to volunteer for the air force, and be ready to answer their questions. Ehrenburg had evidently made it his business to find out what these would be. They would ask Victor if he had any air force connections, or any flying experience, and since this was unlikely at his age, he should say he had belonged to a special Boy Scout troop which had done some glider flying. But first he must go to the library and find out as much about gliders as he could. They were also giving preference to people who knew English, so he should get an English phrase book, learn some sentences by heart – words of greeting and a few obvious expressions – and just spout them at the recruiting officer. The chances were that the man probably knew even less English than he did.

Then he came to the most important point. 'You're a Jew, and some of these Poles are very anti-Semitic. They see this air force unit as an élite formation, and they're unlikely to take many Jews. So you'll have to change your name. Otherwise, they might tumble to it straight away.'

Victor did exactly as Ehrenburg told him, and it worked. Within a few months he was in England, with a brand-new Polish name, dutifully attending the Catholic church parade every Sunday and stealthily observing his companions to see when they were crossing themselves, so that he might make the right movements at the right time.

'But once you were in England,' Jane said, 'you could have dropped the pretence, couldn't you?'

'That's easier said than done. It's probably difficult for you to imagine the gulf between Pole and Jew in Poland, Jane. A Polish Jew isn't a Pole, he's a Jew, a lower being, and here was I masquerading as a true-blooded Pole, accepted as such, listening to jokes about Jews and downright obscenities, and remaining silent. You asked about my guilty secret. Well, there it is.'

'Yes, you told me something about it, once, the bare facts, but I didn't understand how difficult it was. So that's what you were running away from?'

'I suppose you could call it that. In a way, I had to change my whole identity, to live a lie, but without the good reason that some of the Jews had in Europe under Hitler. They did this kind of thing to save their lives and those of their families. I suppose I can blame it on my youth, my immaturity, my loneliness. I was on my own, had no one to confess to, no one to ask for advice. And then I got in deeper and deeper. I made up supporting details to strengthen the main story, so that when people were exchanging reminiscences, as we often did in those days, I could speak up with the others. When I was discharged from the air force after the war and joined the BBC, I thought I might somehow shed my false identity, but it didn't work out like that. I'd kept up with the people I'd known in the air force, and made some friends by then, and I decided I couldn't suddenly turn to them and say, "You know, I'm not the person you think I am, because I'm a Jew." You probably think I could have done it quite easily, and maybe you're right. But then you didn't grow up with my experience as a member of an oppressed, despised minority. Experience can enlighten – or blind.'

'No, Dad, I don't condemn you. And I'm glad, very glad, that you're telling me all about it. It means a lot that you're opening up to me like this.'

'It probably helps me more than it helps you. I don't think I've ever talked like this, not even to your mother. I did tell her a little, many years after we got married, and she said, "How awful that you suffered over this all these years." But then she's not Jewish. You're at least half a Jew. She was very sympathetic, but I don't think she quite understood. It didn't matter to her at all that I hadn't said I was Jewish when we got married. But it mattered to me that I hadn't spoken about it either to her or to you and Richard when you were growing up.'

'You did tell us something.'

'Yes, but it wasn't until you were in your early teens – and even then all I said was that my mother was Jewish. Talking about my mother was a deliberate first step in trying to bring out the whole truth, gradually, little by little. I was testing your reactions, Mum's, Richard's . . .'

'Mum was right, it *was* a lot of fuss about nothing, that part of it, at least to us. But what about your own family in Poland?'

'They're dead.'

'Yes, I know about your immediate family, but what about the rest?'

'Every one of them. Mother, father, brother, sister. Uncles, aunts, cousins. Everybody. I tried to track them down after the war. It was no good. Friends of the family, even acquaintances, I couldn't trace a single one. School friends – all gone. I did make contact with a teacher. He'd always said I'd go a long way, only he didn't know which way, to the good or to the bad. It was a family joke. But he wasn't Jewish. The Jews were all dead. . . .' He paused. Talking about the dead, about the people nearest to him who were lost in the Holocaust, came too close to his own feelings about death.

'Six million?' Jane prompted him quietly.

'Six million.'

She shut her eyes and said nothing for so long that he assumed she must have fallen asleep. She must be exhausted after such a long talk. Victor was rather relieved. It was a painful subject even now. He gently released her hand and walked to the window. When he turned back, her eyes were on him, wide open.

'That's what you've been running away from, Dad,' she said softly. 'The six million.'

He thought about it. 'I suppose I was.'

There was another silence, and then Jane said very gently, 'You still are.'

He stared at her angrily. 'But I'm not, Jane. I'm not making a secret of it any more, you know that. It's all in the history of the *Guardian*, you said that yourself. And I certainly take every opportunity now to make it clear that I'm a Jew. What do you mean, I'm still running away from it?'

But Jane wasn't ready to answer that one yet. She was very tired, yet still refused to give up. It was obviously important to her to have it out with him. She pressed him to talk more about his past – which was part of her past, too.

So he talked about the camps in Russia again. Two million people had been deported to Siberia at the beginning of the war when Stalin had first 'liberated' the eastern half of Poland and mounted a vast police operation to remove all the Poles, Jews, and Ukrainians who were likely to resist.

Young men were rounded up in police raids, families were roused in the middle of the night and loaded into cattle trucks. After as much as a month in a locked truck, they would be set down somewhere in the Siberian wilderness and told to make a new life there. Not everybody even survived the journey.

He spoke about the millions of slave labourers from Russia, Poland, the other countries conquered by Hitler, who were moved around Europe by the Germans and then left stranded in the West, fearing to return to countries taken over by the Communists.

He wasn't just rambling. He was trying to put her own life in historical perspective, to conjure up for her the suffering and the sacrifice and the toll exacted by the war, the movement of millions of people across borders, the separations, the reunions, the heartache and the joy – and, yes, she had made him talk about the dying. The dying he had seen in the Russian camps. The men and women of the Resistance in western Europe just wiped out. The pilots in the Battle of Britain, young and vibrant in the day, dying in the night. The armies moving across Europe, leaving a trail of destruction behind them, the countless dead, so many, so young, as young as she, often younger ... He hoped that this would somehow make it easier for her to accept her own death, put it into some kind of human context for her.

'Six million,' Jane said again.

Were they at cross-purposes? Why did she keep coming back to the six million, to his own life, his own past? At first the reason for her dogged persistence eluded him, but in the end he recognised the pattern. She had set out, as in so many of their other talks, to help him come to terms with what was happening to her. But he could do this only if he first came to terms with himself. He had to face the truth about himself, to come out of hiding. She was using her death to ask questions and to get at the truth of his life in a way she could never have done before. He would not have let her.

She knew that throughout her illness he had avoided the real issue because he could not come to grips with the question of dying: he could not come to terms with her death because he hadn't been able to face the prospect of his own.

He had been running away from it ever since the war when he first denied his Jewishness, his kinship with the six million. But she had led him, step by step, to confront the truth.

'You wanted to learn my guilty secret. Now you know.'

She looked up at him sympathetically. 'It was you who needed to know it, Dad.'

At last Victor was free to talk about it. He no longer pleaded his youth and immaturity. Now he recognised his real motive. During the war, so long as Hitler remained undefeated, he was afraid there was always the chance he might be captured by the Germans and killed if he was identified as a Jew. After the war, when the first detailed accounts of the horrors were published, when he saw the first pictures of the skin-and-bone bodies heaped in the concentration camps, he thought not only of the past but also of the future. If it happened once, it could happen again. Better safe than sorry. He had no family ties, no links to his past, no home to go back to – nothing that made it necessary for him to resume his identity. So he stayed as he was.

'It isn't just that I lived a lie all those years. It's that I didn't admit it even to myself. Well, I have now, Jane.' He looked at her. 'Thanks to you.'

Jane returned his look as if to ask, did he really mean it? Then she smiled at him with a satisfied expression. She had obviously succeeded. Finally she could rest. She dozed off, leaving Victor still thinking about their conversation. She had shown him something he had never reasoned out for himself: that he was very afraid of dying, and that so long as he remained afraid for himself, he would be afraid for her. But she could retain her serenity about her own death only if she could make him share in it. At last he was no longer afraid, because he had faced the truth.

Chapter 12

The next morning we were in the hospice lounge when a smartly dressed woman, obviously a volunteer, came to tell us that a church service would be starting in a few minutes. 'Some of our visitors like to attend with the patients. Would you care to join us?'

'No, thank you very much,' Rosemary said politely.

When she told Jane about it, her daughter pulled a face. 'That's one event I don't mind missing today.'

Dorothy, one of the nurses, who was washing her, looked up. 'Why, Jane, aren't you religious?'

'Far from it. I'm an atheist.'

'Me too!' Dorothy said quickly. 'I'm glad you're open about it. We had one man here who felt terribly guilty. He was surprised when I told him I wasn't religious either, and talking about it seemed to help him forget his guilt.'

'I don't see anything to feel badly about. I just came to the conclusion that there wasn't a God,' Jane said.

'And you don't mind people knowing?'

'It doesn't come out unless you know people fairly well. A lot of them are shocked, and I've known some who thought it was downright evil not to believe in God.'

Dorothy laughed. 'My husband thinks it's arrogant to boast about being an atheist. But I believe one should be honest. We brought our children up to make their own choice when they were old enough.'

'Mum and Dad did that for me, too.'

Jane closed her eyes as if she had talked enough, but later she discussed it with Rosemary.

'I can't believe in any form of life after death although I've tried hard enough, just as I tried to believe in God, but I simply can't.'

'I believe in some kind of recycling process,' Rosemary said.

'Nothing in life is wasted, at least not in the physical world. I don't like the expression "spiritual", it's too loaded for me, but for want of a better word, I feel that the spiritual part of us is indestructible and emerges again in some form. I believe nothing is wasted there, either.'

'I don't think there's anything at all.'

'Just blank?' Rosemary asked. She thought it must be difficult to contemplate such complete emptiness.

'Just nothing,' Jane repeated. Her tone was flat, without emotion.

'It would be comforting to be able to believe in God,' Rosemary said. 'I think it must be a great source of strength to many people.'

'I think so, too,' Jane said calmly. 'I do envy people with that certainty. It must be terrific to have a sense of being supported, with a nice, safe pattern to follow.'

'On the other hand,' Rosemary said, 'something like this is easier to bear – for me, anyway, when you can feel that the course of events isn't being directed from on high, but is completely impersonal, something that just happens. I don't feel it's a question of malice. I believe that ill fortune just hits us, rather than being a punishment for bad behaviour or for not praying often or sincerely enough.'

Jane agreed. 'Wouldn't it be grim to contemplate a universal God arranging everything so that only certain people had it good? Awful to think you only got rewarded if you kept up a continual request for favoured treatment and behaved according to protocol.' She smiled. 'Do you remember when things were really bad early in my illness, and so many people said they were praying for me? More people than I'd ever have expected . . .' her smile broadened as she enjoyed a private joke. 'I used to think sometimes that the reason I wasn't getting any better was precisely because all these people were praying for me!'

Rosemary laughed. 'Yes, I can imagine God saying in answer to their prayers, "No, not that one, not on any account!" It's a terrible impression of a vengeful and rather petty Almighty.'

'Of course, one never knows for sure, but I'm pretty certain there's just nothing,' Jane reiterated.

Victor came in just in time to hear this last remark and wondered whether she was in fact wavering in her atheism. Was she thinking that the time had come to take out an insurance policy?

He remembered how she had believed very strongly in childhood that religion would be the core of her life. She was about ten at the time. She read whatever she could find about Jesus – there wasn't much at home, but she brought books from school. She prayed long and hard, and attended class at a local Protestant church to learn about the Christian faith. She listened, asked questions, and apparently found what she was told acceptable and satisfying. She decided to join the church. Then, a few days before the christening ceremony, she suddenly announced she had changed her mind. We insisted that she carry out her commitment and go through with the ceremony; it was too late to cancel. We didn't ask for her reason. A crisis of faith seemed unlikely in a ten year old. She must learn to keep her commitments, that was what mattered. Jane protested vigorously, but we were firm.

On the morning of the christening she was silent and sullen. She went through the motions at church and then returned home. She never attended a service again. We had often wondered guiltily whether it was our insistence on the christening that had swung her so sharply and completely away from religion. Was it conceivable that she might now revert to her early faith?

Victor felt himself on tricky ground. It was of no account to him at that moment whether there was a God or not; what was important was that if Jane wanted to find God now, she should be helped to do so. He thought he shouldn't approach the subject directly. It would be best to get Jane to recall her childhood experience, perhaps to relive it.

'We've managed to sort out some of our early disagreements,' he began. 'But there was one fight when I behaved particularly badly.'

'Now you make *me* feel guilty,' she said with a grin, 'talking about your guilt. That's not the object of the exercise. You're supposed to be making me feel good!'

'Will it help if I tell you I'm sorry for something we did when you were ten?'

'It depends . . .'

He recalled the drama of her christening. But he dwelt most on how completely she had become absorbed in religion at the beginning, on the joy it had given her.

'When I was growing up,' he said, 'I promised myself that if I ever had children, I'd never treat them as badly as my parents behaved to me. I remember swearing that adults never understand, but I would be different.'

'Every child does that, Dad.'

'Did you?'

'Oh yes, many times.'

'Were we as bad as that to you?'

'Now you're fishing.'

'Was that one of the times, the christening?'

'I don't remember,' she said quickly. Her tone and expression made it quite clear she didn't want to talk about it.

Later, Victor tried to approach the subject from a different angle, recalling how he, too, had lost his faith at about the same age. He had begun to doubt God's existence, and had then challenged Him: 'If You're there, You'll punish me for such sinful thoughts.' When no punishment followed, he declared himself an atheist. 'But that was rather childish,' he admitted.

It wasn't unique, Jane said, warming to the subject. She told him how her grandmother, Rosemary's mother, who had died when Jane was seventeen, had decided to find out about the mighty and terrible God for herself. 'She went and stood in the middle of a very large field, and said "Damn", but very softly, because she'd been told that God heard and saw everything and no sin went unpunished. She stood there, waiting to be struck down by a thunderbolt. Nothing happened. She said, "Damn", again, louder this time, in case God had been busy with something else and had missed it. Again nothing happened, so she shouted it aloud:

"Damn!" More silence. That convinced her that God couldn't exist. She told me it was all rather an anticlimax.'

This was the opening Victor wanted. 'But Granny gave me the impression of being a religious person.'

'She didn't think much of the clergy.'

'Which was just as well. She had no strong feelings about a church wedding for your mother, and my Jewish God might have taken offence at that.'

'Yes, Granny worked out her own brand of religion, which excluded the church and priests. She believed in the precepts of the Bible, if not the story.'

'I think she found it very comforting. Many people do.'

'Yes, I would, too, if I *could* believe.'

Victor pressed on. 'But I don't see much difference between your way of life, your ethics, and those of the Christian religion, or any other religion for that matter. In a way, you're a very religious person, Jane. Not unlike Granny, and she regained her early faith, as so many other people do.'

'No, Dad, it's no good. I can't believe if it's not in me. I know you're trying to help, but I can do without that kind of assistance.'

That same morning, Rosemary fetched herself something to eat in the staff kitchen, which was also available to relatives. She sat down beside a man in brown overalls who was finishing a cup of coffee. 'Excuse me,' he asked, 'how did your daughter sleep?'

'Very well, thanks,' Rosemary said, touched by this friendly interest from a stranger.

'I was there when they brought her in.' He looked at her sadly. 'I thought about her all night.'

'You work here?'

'That's right. I'm kept busy moving stores, helping move patients.'

He must be the porter, she thought, but he didn't sound like one, more like a partner with pride in his firm, as he told her: 'I'm happier working here than I've ever been in my life before. When I leave, I've done what's a worthwhile day's work, and it's real, it's human beings I'm dealing with.'

It was indeed Frank, the porter. He visited all the patients every day, stopping to talk to those who felt like it, offering to run errands and finding out if there was anything he could do to make the day pleasanter for them. Later, Jane was to have long talks with him.

Jane meanwhile was turning down a bath. She hadn't improved that much.

'We have special apparatus here that lifts you into the bath and raises you out again when we've washed you,' Julia told her. 'You won't have to move or do anything.'

Jane looked regretful. Bathing had been one of life's pleasures for her. 'I'm sorry . . . I don't think I can handle it. . . .'

'Don't let it worry you. I'll pop in again in about an hour. You may feel more rested then.'

But the answer was still no. 'I'm sorry. I really can't.'

'Then we'll give you a blanket bath instead.'

Jane relaxed.

Rosemary returned, grateful that Julia had been so under-standing and that Jane hadn't needed her support. It had been very different in the hospital, she told Julia. 'We often felt that some of the doctors didn't really believe Jane felt as much pain as she said she did.'

'It's not easy to understand what another person is suffering,' Julia said.

'Jane's face was always bright and healthy-looking. She didn't look seriously ill. You couldn't actually *see* her pain. I kept telling people she was far sicker than she looked, but they probably thought I was just being over-protective.'

A faint voice came from the bed. 'Be fair, Mum. Most of the nurses were very good to me. They were often just too busy when I desperately needed someone to talk to, especially at night.'

'You won't be alone here,' said Julia firmly. 'I remember a quote from somewhere that stuck in my mind because it sums up what I think about pain. "Pain is what the patient says he feels".'

A group of Jane's friends came from London to see her. There was Michael, Jane's old love, and Kate, with her vivid red curls and lively face – both had been among Jane's most frequent visitors. The other two, Ruth and Dick, she had known only since her illness. She would probably find four of them too much on one afternoon, they explained, but they had wanted to come. Victor warned them they must be careful not to tire her. She didn't have much more time. Nobody knew how long – weeks rather than months, according to the doctors.

The four friends, all about Jane's age, were appalled. *Weeks* rather than months? They couldn't absorb emotionally what they had known for a long time intellectually. They had been only too ready to deceive themselves; they had come to cheer her up, as they'd done so often before, in so many different hospitals. One went to a hospital to be cured. Jane was their contemporary. To think of her death made them feel mortal, too.

'She knows it won't be long now,' Victor explained, 'and she's quite reconciled to it. But she needs your help. Don't pretend that nothing's happening. If she wants to talk about her death, let her. Don't deny it.'

Michael was the first of the four to go in. He refused to accept Victor's prognosis. He was still determined that Jane should fight for her life. He worked again, as he did when he used to visit her in the hospital, to steer her towards the world of the living – ignoring the signs, her great weakness, her indifference to his conversation, and what Victor had told him of her rapidly deteriorating condition. He couldn't accept that she was going to die of cancer so soon.

He talked to her of politics, and of his own involvement in a strike at a local factory, where passions had risen so high that the police had been brought in to control the pickets. Once he and Jane had been politically involved together. Surely she would be interested in his story. He explained that as a local Labour Party member he had been asked to support the pickets, but fighting had broken out at the factory gates. The police made many arrests, and he too had been detained.

Jane didn't respond, but Michael persisted, trying hard to

get her attention. He gave a blow-by-blow account of the fight at the picket line and of his arrest. He told of his anxieties about the forthcoming court case. It seemed as if she could hardly hear what he was saying. Perhaps it was the dope, he thought.

Victor's arrival with lunch was a welcome diversion. He could see that Michael and his daughter were not on the same wavelength, and tried to find a way to bring them together again. He remembered them as young lovers at the university, each so absorbed in the other that the rest of the world hardly existed for them. He handed Michael a plate. 'Would you help Jane with this?'

Very carefully, Michael fed her small teaspoonfuls from the plate, trying to persuade her to eat. But Jane refused to make the effort. Again he attempted to catch her interest, to involve her in the outside world. He told her how worried he was that a police record might harm his career. She failed to respond.

'Come on, now,' he urged her. 'Have another bite. It'll help you to get better.'

'No.' Her voice was weak but the tone was final. 'I don't want any.'

Victor's intervention hadn't helped. Now he must extricate Michael without hurting his feelings. He told him that Jane must have a rest, then it would be Kate's turn. Michael came away painfully aware of his failure to make contact with Jane, but still hoping it was only a temporary setback. Perhaps she would be in better shape when he returned in a few days.

Kate saw immediately how much weaker Jane was, but she greeted her warmly, hiding her shock. Dorothy brought in the mashed banana and milk Jane liked, and Jane introduced the two women, an old friend and a new one. 'I'm proud of my friends, Dorothy,' she said. 'I can see you've cause to be,' Dorothy responded. 'There's a whole bunch of them in the hall waiting to see you. Now, would you like a hot drink or some ice cream?'

'No, thanks very much. But I did eat some of my beans.' Jane spoke as if she'd done enough. She didn't want the banana, but she didn't like to hurt Dorothy's feelings. When

Dorothy left the room, she asked Kate to put the food aside; she might be able to eat it later.

'How are you feeling? Any better?' Kate asked quietly.

'Not really. The pain was pretty awful when they brought me here, but it's not so bad now.' She went on almost casually, 'I don't think it's going to be long before I die.' Then, before Kate could answer, she asked: 'Who else came today? Michael would only talk about his strike.'

'Dick and Ruth are here, but they told me to tell you it's all right if you're too tired. We came to find out how you were and if you felt like seeing us . . .' she broke off, then began again, trying to sound more everyday, more normal. 'Nice place here, isn't it? So friendly. . . .'

Jane's attention had wandered. Now she focused on the moment again. 'Did you say Ruth? I'd love to see her, could she come in too?'

Ruth, a comparative newcomer to Jane's circle of friends, walked in uneasily, not sure whether she should intrude. As she took Jane's hand, she noticed how fragile it had become, almost too frail to stand the pressure of her own healthy fingers. She wondered how much Jane knew about her slowly developing relationship with Michael. Ruth had sensed many times over the past few months that Jane was aware of what was happening even before they were themselves. She held the thin hand shyly for a moment, then released it.

'Please don't take your hand away, Ruth. Tell me what's been happening.'

As she talked, Ruth began to relax. She took turns with Kate, feeding the mashed banana to Jane with a teaspoon. 'It's a bit like feeding a baby,' Jane remarked with some embarrassment, gesturing weakly to the huge white napkin Dorothy had wrapped round her neck and shoulders to protect her from drips and splashes. They lifted her head slightly; it didn't seem to hurt. They took a long time over the job, but Ruth noticed how little Jane actually ate.

'What I'd really like is not more food, but someone to move my legs. They feel very strange these days.'

Her feet were even weaker than her hands. Kate tried to rub some life into them.

Jane thanked her, adding hesitantly: 'I'm so happy that I

have such good friends. You must think I sound sloppy today, but that's the way I feel.'

Kate was deeply moved. Jane had managed to put a wealth of meaning into a few words. She was too weak to say much, but her brief remark recalled their happy times together, how close they had become, and seemed a reminder of the change that was occurring in Jane. Yes, it did sound sentimental, quite unlike the Jane she had known; but then, she had a right to express her feelings.

Kate fought to control herself. 'Let's all have a cigarette,' she said.

The three women smoked together. Kate and Ruth were aware how strong and healthy they must look to Jane, but as time went by her attitude helped them to forget the contrast. She had a look of complete serenity which, although it was hard to understand, calmed them. Only then did Jane say quietly, almost with contentment: 'The doctors think it won't be long before I die.'

Kate was convinced Jane wasn't just pretending for their sake. She thought, *Jane really means it*, she's telling us she can take it – but can I?

Ruth concentrated on holding the ashtray to catch the ash that spilled from Jane's cigarette, sagging forgotten between limp fingers. When Jane did remember, she had difficulty controlling it as she lifted it to and from her mouth. Finally she dozed off with the cigarette still in her hands. Both friends wondered what to do. Let her sleep, Ruth signalled. Kate gently eased the cigarette out of Jane's fingers.

Soon Jane opened her eyes again. Slowly she raised her hand towards her mouth, as if continuing the motion begun when she had dropped off, and seemed surprised to find it empty. 'Where's my cigarette?'

For Ruth, this was the moment when she could take no more. She got up to go.

If Jane noticed her distress, she gave no sign. She just said, 'I'm glad I knew you, Ruth. I'd like to see you again. If I can't make it, then I'd like to say goodbye . . .'

Ruth kissed her quickly and left the room. She realised now that Jane sensed how things were between her and Michael, and that she was happy about it.

Left alone with Jane, Kate had to struggle not to break down. When Jane, speaking very deliberately, offered Kate one of her shawls, her friend couldn't maintain her careful casualness. 'No, no, you really don't need to think about that,' she protested.

'You always liked the material,' Jane persisted, 'remember?' Kate couldn't answer. She wondered how Jane, so close to dying, could think of giving presents.

Rosemary looked in at this point to make sure Jane wasn't getting too tired and heard the conversation. 'I think Jane would really like you to have the shawl, Kate. We've been talking a lot about the presents she wants to give her friends. It means a great deal to her.'

Fighting to control herself, Kate managed to say: 'Well, in that case – I'd love it. It's beautiful. Thank you, Jane.'

When Jane's friends left the hospice, they went to a nearby pub on the river, too upset to go home. It was a grey day, cold and oppressive. The gloomy weather accentuated the sadness of the parting. They talked about Jane, wanting to save her, to protect her. Each of them knew that whatever they had given her in the past, either separately or together, could never have been enough to prove their love for her. Now it was too late to do any more. They felt totally helpless.

Jane, too, was thinking sadly of her friends, especially Michael. She alternated between irritation that he had talked only about his strike when they had so little time together and acute anxiety that he was in real trouble.

'Michael kept on and on about the pickets,' she muttered to her mother. 'As if I care.'

Then again, after an interval of dozing: 'Mum, I wish you'd find out what's happening at Michael's house. I'm worried. I can't help feeling he's in danger. He may be arrested.'

'Try not to worry, darling. He's on bail and you can be absolutely sure he won't risk getting arrested again.'

'But you don't realise what it's like, Mum. There are people who live in the area who don't like them. They might make trouble.'

'What kind of trouble? It's a very quiet neighbourhood.' Rosemary tried to get Jane's fears out into the open.

'There could be a brick through the window, something like that. I've got this feeling that bad things are happening.'

Jane calmed down only when Richard told her he had phoned Michael and all was well. She knew Richard would give her the unvarnished truth, good or bad.

The rest of the family went back to Dairy Cottage, and Rosemary was left alone with Jane until the following evening. After they had gone, Rosemary was overcome by a sense of isolation and depression. Richard was soon to return to America, and the family was divided about this decision. The hospice, normally so homelike, seemed totally deserted; the other visitors had long since gone home and the nurses were all attending to the patients. She was concerned that she would find it difficult to hide her low spirits from Jane. But she needn't have worried. Jane was talking happily to Sarah, a different nurse, who was busy making her as comfortable as possible for the night.

When Jane was settled. Sarah turned to her mother. Had she enough bedding – another pillow, maybe? Would she like a hot drink? She must be sure to help herself to anything she wanted from the kitchen in the night, Sarah insisted.

From the room next door came the sound of voices: 'Would you like sherry tonight, Mr. Dick, as a change from your usual?'

'No thanks, Sister. I'll stick to my brandy.'

It sounded more like a nightcap at home than the distribution of drugs from the late night medicine trolley.

We had got through another day, and Jane was comfortable and content.

Chapter 13

Unknown to Rosemary, the hospice staff worried about her attitude. Adela had reported a seemingly casual remark of Rosemary's while the two of them were exercising Jane's legs to relax her body: 'Now that I know how, I'll be able to do this for you when we go home, Jane.' Adela was distressed. Didn't she realise Jane was never going home again? There was a danger this might influence Jane's attitude, too, so that she would be less ready to accept her death when it came. The nurses decided to find out what Rosemary's thoughts really were. It was Sarah who drew her aside. 'How do you feel about Jane's illness now?' she asked, looking at her intently.

Rosemary knew at once what she meant. 'I've known for a long time that Jane hadn't much longer to live,' she replied without hesitation. 'She always seemed more ill than people thought. I've watched her grow steadily weaker.' Rosemary still half-hoped Jane might die at home, but she had no doubt that her death was very near.

There was no need for either of them to say any more. Suddenly, Sarah smiled. 'She is a smashing girl!' she said. Rosemary smiled back gratefully, deeply touched. They had communicated far more than the mere words they used. This capacity for quick, easy understanding was part of the hospice atmosphere, and Jane had come to share in it, too. All her life she had been slow to get to know people, wary of lowering her own defences, inclined to keep strangers at a distance. Now she was on close terms with everyone who came into her bedroom, responding rapidly to the warmth of the hospice.

Sometimes she was ready for serious conversations, but she also enjoyed the small talk that can be so comforting to sick people who need to communicate but aren't always up to more intense discussions. The hospice staff knew that minor matters are important to the bedridden.

Jane had always been fastidious, relishing the sensation of cleanliness; but a blanket bath, when she was washed in bed with the minimum of movement, was the closest she could get to the joy she used to derive from relaxing in a tub. She told Dorothy how much she liked the soft feel of the sponge and asked her to take her time over it. Sensitive to her mood, Dorothy lingered over the task. She had never owned a natural sponge herself, and commented with surprise on its light touch. This was enough for Jane. As soon as Rosemary came in, Jane said: 'Mum, when you go shopping, could you take my money and get a proper sponge for Dorothy? A really nice one – she's been so good to me. I'd like her to have something she'll use every day.' Jane was still thinking of giving presents, and she asked Rosemary to make pots for all the staff when she got back to her work.

On the other side of the wall an old man began to cough, noisily and painfully. Jane stirred uneasily and finally said with annoyance: 'The pain's getting pretty bad. Could I have another injection?'

Sarah came immediately. 'Of course you can have an injection if you need it,' she said. 'But let's try and see if we can't make you comfortable first. That would ease the pain a lot. It's some time since we turned you. We'll move you onto your right side.'

She asked Rosemary if she would help.

'Of course, if you'll tell me what to do. I'm a bit afraid of hurting her.' It was very difficult for Rosemary to handle her daughter's body now. In the past weeks, when her efforts to wash or lift Jane had caused extra suffering, Rosemary had felt an inept nurse. But hospice workers are trained to encourage reluctant relatives to help.

'Now,' said Sarah, 'I'll take her body. Just push your arms right under the legs, as I'm doing with her back, and then we'll gently ease her over in one. Right? Ready?'

Jane lay atop their four arms, quite helpless. Sarah had

arranged her legs so that they were slightly bent at the knees and hips to reduce tension on the stomach muscles, for that was the area of great pain. Her body's reactions to every movement had been carefully noted and thoroughly discussed at the staff's daily conference. Sarah knew where the cancer hurt most. As she turned Jane over, she avoided provoking the additional pain that twisting or stress on the spine would cause. Since the spine often aches when one is lying in bed for long periods, Sarah packed pillows against Jane's back to provide support and to give her confidence that her body wouldn't slip to a less comfortable position. Helpless patients can worry about slipping, and the hospice staff was alert to these fears.

But Jane wasn't comfortable yet. Sarah persisted in her efforts to find a relaxed position, lowering first the head of the bed, then the foot, asking her at intervals if she felt more at ease. Jane became embarrassed that she always answered no, but Sarah waved the apologies aside. 'It's no trouble,' she said. 'We've got plenty of time.'

Rosemary helped to lift Jane over until she lay on her left side again. Once more Sarah packed her body with cushions, easing the pressure here, supporting it there, rearranging the limbs with infinite patience.

At last Jane smiled. 'That's much better. I might get to sleep now.'

But the pain returned, and Rosemary had to go looking for a nurse again. Sarah came back promptly. The hospice was determined to control her suffering. She gave Jane an injection immediately.

When Patricia came on duty later, Rosemary was worried Jane might get upset again. But the two were soon friends.

When Jane arrived at the hospice four days before, Patricia had been well aware of her hostility. Now she found that Jane was no longer a bundle of pain. A conversation started up when Patricia commented on Jane's hair as she brushed it. It was still thick and shining, she said, in spite of the treatments.

'I was scared of losing it all with chemotherapy,' Jane responded. 'I used to count the hairs in my comb every day. I thought I was going to look like a scarecrow. I suppose it's silly, but I'd have been very embarrassed to have people see me like that.'

It could have been something in Pat's manner – perhaps the very directness and briskness that had irritated her the first day – that now made Jane think she could put the question, 'I wonder how long it will be before I die?' It came easily, naturally.

'I don't expect it'll be long now,' Pat said, in an equally matter-c　act way. For the moment, that seemed to be all Jane wanted. Pat was brushing the hair away from her face. 'You really do look very beautiful, you know.'

'That's hard to believe.' Jane giggled, pleased in spite of herself. She had always done what she could to look as good as possible.

'No, you do look lovely. So serene. I thought so when you first came in – how lovely you looked in spite of the pain.'

'Really?' she sounded sceptical. 'I haven't seen myself for ages, and then I looked pretty foul.'

It hadn't occurred to anyone at Dairy Cottage to offer her a mirror. When Jane went to the bathroom, she didn't stop to look at herself. The pain caused by the movement had made her want to get back to bed as quickly as possible. But the hospice nurses knew how much their looks mattered to the patients, old and young, men and women. That was one reason why the list of things a patient should bring to the hospice included a hand mirror.

'Where's your mirror, Jane? You must see for yourself.' Patricia rummaged in the locker beside the bed, then held the glass up so she could look easily. 'Can you see properly? It is such a tiny mirror.'

'Could you bring it closer? I can't see very well.' Jane studied her face silently, then she said thoughtfully, 'I hope I die looking like this. I don't want to end up looking hideous. Sounds silly, doesn't it?' She made a face. 'It shouldn't matter what you look like.'

'I don't think it's silly at all, Jane. You'll be lovely, I promise you.'

Jane took another look at the mirror and rested her head on the pillow. She was smiling.

Among the friends Jane had asked to see was Ann, whom she had first met when they taught at the same school. Ann arrived while Dr. Murray was with Jane and Rosemary was in the nurse's kitchen making bread. It was one of Jane's favourite foods, and she had taught Rosemary how to do it. The kitchen smelled strongly of yeast. Ann spoke quickly, as if embarrassed.

'You know, when I got Richard's message that Jane would like to see me I had no idea – I hadn't heard anything at all about her – I was a bit shattered . . .' She paused, as if unsure how to go on. 'I was rather afraid to meet you, but it's a relief to see you're managing. One never knows how people will be affected and I didn't know you at all, only what Jane told me.'

'Yes, it has been hard.' Rosemary kneaded the dough vigorously. 'But Jane's happy now, you'll see that, and everyone's marvellous to us. We've been made to feel at home.'

'And the nurses don't mind you being here all the time?'

'Nobody says anything, no matter how many of Jane's friends turn up. Today, Monday, is officially a non-visiting day, but it's meant to give the patients' families a rest as much as the patients themselves. Sometimes it's difficult for people to travel long distances every day. That way those who need a day to themselves have an excuse, and there don't have to be hurt feelings.'

'I can see they think of everything.'

'But if people want to visit, the nurses like it.' She told Ann about Arloc, and how the hospice staff had made him welcome.

'Everyone seems so – well, unbrisk, if one could use such a word,' Ann said. 'I remember when my mother was dying a few years ago, it was very different. They had such strict rules – she was in hospital, of course. She was much too ill to be looked after at home. I wanted my daughter Judy, she was ten, to see her grandmother before she died. But when I asked permission to bring her into the ward, Sister said absolutely not. It would damage the child to see someone she loved in such a state. So I just said: "Look, I'm sorry, but I'm going to bring my daughter here to see her grandmother whatever you say." And I did. Judy told me afterwards that seeing someone dying wasn't nearly as bad as she'd imagined it might. She'd had all sorts of horrible fears about it, and then everything was quite simple and easy for her.'

They were interrupted by Dr. Murray's arrival. 'Patricia said I'd find you here . . .'

Ann went off to see Jane. 'Dr. Murray,' Rosemary began, 'I wanted to ask you about something that's worrying Jane. She's forcing herself to drink even though she doesn't want to.' She explained that Jane had been warned at the hospital that if she didn't take enough liquid she would need another saline drip. 'She really hated it.'

'That won't happen here. We don't feed intravenously,' he reassured her. 'You remember our discussion about nerve blocks? I've been talking to Jane about blocking off her nerves to deal with the pain she still feels. But it's early days yet.'

'She does complain of pain sometimes.'

'She's moving more now and the movements produce pain. I explained this, and she appeared to accept it. If we do block off her nerves to deal with the pain, it's simply a matter of giving an injection of a nerve poison like phenol. This would knock out the nerve fibres for a time.'

'We were worried about her having to be moved. She still has nightmares and asks: "Where do we go when we have to leave?" She needs to feel secure.'

'It can be done in her room,' he reassured her.

There was something else bothering Rosemary. 'Richard has to go back to America on Wednesday. He's spending tonight with Jane, then Arloc will come over tomorrow to see her. It'll be their last day here.'

'That will be very difficult for her,' Dr. Murray agreed. 'We'll do what we can to help her through it.'

Rosemary thought of Arloc and his easy, natural manner with Jane. The boy had never treated her as a being apart because she had cancer; her illness had been no source of embarrassment to him. 'She'll miss Arloc as well as Richard,' she said. 'Yesterday he just sat holding her hand and neither of them needed to say anything.'

Meanwhile, Ann and Jane were chatting. 'Shouldn't you be in school?' Jane asked.

'I had a free afternoon. When the others heard I was coming here, they helped me get off early. I didn't expect to see you looking so bright.'

'They give me injections whenever I need them and I'm fine. I still get nightmares, though. Last night I was in an Italian brothel and furious that the Mafia were getting all the profits. Mum said I tried hard to persuade her we should escape. I must've been pretty scared.' She yawned. 'It was a tiring night. I'm sorry – I do get very sleepy.'

'I have the whole afternoon, so if you want to drop off, feel free,' Ann assured her.

'Did Richard tell you everything?'

'Yes, he did.'

'He told you I was going to die?'

'Yes,' Ann answered without hesitation. 'Are you frightened?' The words came out naturally, but even as she spoke, she thought this was a silly question. Jane's answer made her realise that it hadn't been tactless after all.

'I *was* frightened,' Jane stressed. 'I'm not now, not any more.'

Ann felt that all the barriers were down. The restraints common in a conversation between people not entirely intimate no longer existed. They were closer than ever before.

'I seem to have slipped down in the bed. Would you mind giving me a lift up? The nurses do so much, I hate to keep interrupting them for little things.'

'Of course I'd like to help you,' Ann said hesitantly, 'but I'm a bit scared of hurting you.'

Jane said she should try, so Ann put her arms beneath her friend's shoulders and pulled her up in the bed. They both giggled at Ann's clumsiness as she moved the limp body. How soft it was, thought Ann. Soft and limp, as if she had no bones left, no muscles, no strength.

'Did you mind touching me?' Jane asked her. 'Some people find it embarrassing, especially when one is naked?'

'No, of course not.'

'That's one of the really great things about this place. They don't get in a state over silly little things. Here they treat me like a human being all the time, not just when they feel like it.'

Jane looked so virginal and good, Ann thought. Her expression was almost elated. When she talked about dying, it seemed as if she welcomed death, and not merely as an escape. But they spoke easily of other things, too. 'Do you get many birds coming to the bird table?' Ann asked, peering out of the window.

'It was there when we came and Arloc filled it with food. I think they moved it nearer to the window, but I still can't see very well.'

'There's a bird on it now. I think it's a greenfinch.'

'Mum says he keeps the other birds from feeding.'

Jane lay back and her attention drifted. Perhaps she wanted to sleep. Ann left soon. She decided she should share this experience with the class that Jane had taught. She would try to describe Jane's feelings about dying.

Ann's visit had made it possible for Rosemary to get away from the hospice for a short time. Sue, an old friend who lived nearby, took her for a walk in the brilliant June sunshine. Rosemary picked some poppies, remembering how Jane loved their deep scarlet colour. As the stalks broke, the familiar acrid scent rose up. This would be a far richer experience for Jane now that her sight was failing. The smell would bring back memories of sights and sounds, and enrich what time she had left.

Together Sue and Rosemary walked round searching for smells, and not just the sweet ones. Jane had never been a 'sweet' person, she had loved unusual tangy scents – that of dandelions, for example. They could find no dandelion flowers, but the plant itself was there and its leaves carried the strong pungent odour. Herb Robert grew nearby, too, the strong smell of its seeds surprising in such a modest and fragile plant. They found other flowers and leaves whose names they didn't know. They picked from every plant in sight, then tested each for smell before adding it to the bunch or rejecting it. Even strong, slightly unpleasant odours, like that of the flower called stinking mayweed, would be worth experiencing one more time. Clover flowers, sweet and slightly dusty, would bring back the most typical scent of summer.

They carried their bunch of 'smells' back to Jane and held each flower, each leaf, in turn to her nose. She sniffed deeply, her eyes shut, a smile of pleasure on her lips as she tried to identify them one by one.

Later in the evening Sue returned with a branch of orange blossom, and the vivid smell filled the room. She also brought a bunch of herbs. As she held them for Jane, she rubbed each herb, releasing the aroma. Many of these were herbs that Jane had used to flavour her cooking. Some of them grew in her own garden. She sniffed slowly, taking a deep breath each time, and waiting before going on to the next: lemon thyme, marjoram, bergamot, tarragon, rosemary, mint ... Each carried many memories. It was as if she were saying goodbye to old friends with whom she had shared good times.

Chapter 14

Victor was very angry at the thought that Richard would be returning to Boston in two days. Here was Richard's sister on her death bed, and he couldn't wait to get away. Victor didn't put it that way to his son, for he was conscious of the need to avoid family friction at such a time, but he tried to convey his concern.

Richard remained unmoved. He had accomplished what he had come to do: Jane would be well looked after in the hospice. The danger that Rosemary might attempt to cope on her own, and perhaps break down in the process, had been averted. The old conflict between Victor and Jane had been brought to the surface, and they were now talking about their past differences. Above all, Jane knew where she stood. The conspiracy of silence was ended. She had accepted the prospect of dying in a way that he would never have believed possible.

Richard's logic seemed unassailable; Victor tried appealing to his emotions. It was true that Jane had now accepted death, but she might change her mind. Suppose she refused to talk to them again and they needed Richard's help? It was a subtle threat, with a hint of moral blackmail. But Richard felt certain there was no going back now. Lies and deception would not survive in the truthful atmosphere of the hospice – and the truth would help Jane maintain her peace of mind.

Next, Victor appealed to his son's sense of propriety. 'What would people say?' Friends of the family were bound to ask questions; Jane's own friends would be shocked. Why had he left at this crucial time, when the family – any family – ought to be together? They would regard it as desertion, betrayal.

'If that's what they think,' Richard retorted angrily, 'then they're no friends.' He owed them no explanation. His conscience was clear. He knew that what he was doing was right. He wasn't just thinking of himself. Arloc had been missing school, and no one knew how long Jane might live. It could be weeks, even months. If he waited, then the same objections to his departure might be raised at any time in the future. He had obligations on the other side of the Atlantic. Joan had told him he should feel free to stay on, but he had a great deal of work to do which couldn't be put off indefinitely.

'Anyway,' he said, 'I've told Jane I have to go. I've explained why, and she quite agrees.'

Victor didn't utter the words on the tip of his tongue, 'What do you expect her to say?' If Richard had already told Jane, he thought, the damage was beyond repair. He didn't mention to anyone the real reason why he objected to Richard's departure. Deep down, he was terrified that by making it necessary for Jane to say goodbye to him, Richard was compelling her to face the prospect of dying in the starkest, most direct way possible. In these circumstances, the acknowledgement that she would never see him again would mean that, as far as Richard was concerned, she was dying here and now. Should they make her die twice just because Richard wanted to leave?

And there was another even deeper objection which Victor himself was reluctant to acknowledge. The difference between them went back to the original issue that had caused so much heartbreak in the earlier days. Once again the question was whether Jane should be told; but now it arose in a different guise. In opposing Richard's departure, Victor was acting on his old belief that Jane should not be forced to face the prospect of dying. In deciding to leave, Richard was acting out the assumptions underlying his own attitude on this issue, that Jane should be helped to face what was coming. Victor was not bothered by the contradiction inherent in his own attitude. At one moment he was aware that Jane had accepted death, the next moment he refused to act on the assumption that she had done so. For, at the deepest level of all, it was his own fear of dying that caused him to object to Jane being faced with the prospect of death. In spite of all the evidence to the contrary, in spite of his own apparent understanding of Jane's attitude of acceptance, he still couldn't believe that she had come to terms with it. Fearing death himself, he could not easily conceive of anyone who did not fear it.

Meanwhile Jane had asked David Murray how long she would live, as she had asked so many others in recent days, in a way which seemed calculated to let them all know that she was 'ready to go', as one of the nurses put it. To Victor it seemed she had asked virtually everybody except him. He wondered why he had been excluded, but the reason did not occur to him until later, when he finally realised she could not speak to him plainly until she was sure that he, too, had come to terms with death. How, he wondered, could they reassure her that the dying would not take too long? David had now explained to her the medical circumstances which made him think it would be 'weeks rather than months,' but even that, Victor thought, was much longer than she wanted.

Perhaps he ought to find out whether the hospice had a policy on euthanasia. But first he needed to discuss it with Rosemary and Richard. If Richard's travel plans were not changed, he would have to move fast.

'Should I try to talk Richard out of going?' Victor asked Dr. Murray, hoping for an ally.

David wanted to know Richard's reasons, which Victor listed as fully as he could remember them, consciously trying to be fair. He also explained his own attitude. But he didn't reveal his fear that the farewell would shock Jane, that it might seem to her like a rehearsal for her death. He was still unable to acknowledge the contradictions in his own motives. There was his own fear of even the thought of death coupled with his willingness to consider euthanasia.

'Richard's reasons seem valid to me,' David said. Life had to go on, and Richard's obligations to his new family and to his work were no less real because Jane was dying.

'Richard has done his bit,' he added. 'He won't help Jane by staying on.'

'Rosemary seems to think he could even help her by going,' Victor admitted. 'Is it possible that Jane is holding on for Richard, perhaps subconsciously, and that once he's left, she might let go?'

'That's quite possible. It might well help her to let go a little bit more if they say goodbye to each other.'

Victor felt he had been defeated. He couldn't question David's professional judgement. Indeed, he welcomed it, because it absolved him of any responsibility. This was certainly not a good time to have a family argument.

Richard arrived with a huge bunch of flowers. 'Who are these from?' Jane asked, delightedly, as he held it up near the bed so she could smell them and see the colours.

'I don't know,' he said. 'I found them on the path outside Dairy Cottage. There's no more, nothing to say who left them there.' Perhaps it was a neighbour who didn't know what to say.

'They've been picked from somebody's garden,' Rosemary said. 'That's not a flower-shop bunch. I hope we find out who sent them.'

'Put them close where I can smell them . . .'

Richard settled down in the bed next to Jane's. They both fell asleep. Jane woke up for an injection and then she wanted his company. There were things to be said before he left.

'Rich?'

'Yes, what is it?'

'What's the time?'

'Two o'clock.'

'Are you asleep?'

'I'm trying to be. Do you want something?'

'I was having a dream.'

Instantly, he was alert. 'Would you like to tell me about it?'

'You know that Mum and I have talked about scattering my ashes over the garden?'

'Yes.'

She gave a nervous laugh. 'That's what I was dreaming about. A party in the garden. Where the stream runs into the pond. All the people stumbling in the mud, tripping over themselves, scattering my ashes.'

'Is it upsetting you, Jane? There's no need to scatter the ashes unless you want it.'

'Oh, no, I'm not frightened,' she said, guessing his thoughts. 'I rather like the idea of my ashes coming to rest by the stream at Dairy Cottage. Do you remember the day we dug it up and built a dam across it?'

'Not a very good dam. It kept leaking.'

'But it was fun. And it'll be a fun place for my ashes. Not just the stream. The pond. The flower beds. Under the yew trees . . .'

Richard began to fall asleep again. 'Rich?'

'What is it now?' he asked a little testily, trying to suppress his irritation but not succeeding very well.

'Could you get me a cigarette?'

'Are you sure you really want one, Jane?' He felt physically exhausted, emotionally drained.

'Yes, I usually have one at this time, after the injection. It helps me get back to sleep.'

He put the cigarette between her lips and she reached up to it, trying to hold it while he lit a match. But she didn't have a sure grasp and the cigarette slipped out of her mouth.

'Here, let me do it for you,' he said, and puffed on it once or twice to get it going, hating the taste. She looked up at him gratefully and he felt a bit ashamed of himself. She drew on it greedily. Soon a little spur of ash appeared at the end, and hung down precariously.

'Here, Jane, let me knock the ash off,' he said quickly, but her movements were more certain now. She took the cigarette out of her mouth, gave it to him to get rid of the ash, then held her hand out so that he could put it back between her fingers.

Richard was finding it difficult to keep his eyes open. Nora came in to ask if Jane was all right but quickly decided it was Richard who needed help.

'What you need is a cup of strong black coffee.' She was back swiftly with one.

'Room service in the middle of the night,' Richard said to Jane.

'You wouldn't get that in the best hotels – or hospitals. You know, Rich, we might not have come here if it hadn't been for you. When you go back, they'll look after me here. Better, much better, than in hospital. Better than I could have been looked after at home. Mum would have been exhausted in no time. David says it may not be very long now, but they can never be quite sure. I don't want it to be long. It's Dad and Mum I'm worried about, not you. It could be a great shock for them.'

'Don't underestimate them, Jane. You know how strong Mum is when she's decided what's the right thing to do. And Dad's gone through quite a lot himself. He can take it.'

'I don't know. We've talked about his war experiences. Maybe it's helped to bring him round a little.'

The cigarette had gone out; her speech was getting more and more sluggish. She seemed ready to go to sleep, yet she was fighting it. Every now and again, just as Richard's eyes were closing in spite of his determination to keep her company, she would make some inconsequential remark as if she were determined to keep him awake. *She knows it's the last time we'll really be together.* Perhaps she was deliberately trying to prolong it. Yet Richard could not prevent his irritation, though he felt guilty about it.

'I can't see properly, Richard – are you drinking something?'

'The nurse brought me a cup of coffee,' he answered wearily.

'I wonder if perhaps I can have something, too.'

'I'll ask them to make you a drink.'

'No, I don't mean that. You know, I haven't had any food for ages. I think I'm hungry,' she said, pleased at the sensation.

'Well,' he said doubtfully, 'I suppose I could ask.'

'No, that would be giving them too much trouble.'

'They did say, Jane, to tell them any time you wanted anything.'

'All the same, I don't want to overdo it. Maybe I can just have a snack? I'm sure there must be some food here. Mum always has a little something hidden away, just in case.'

Richard began looking around the room, checking the

contents of the shelves and inside the locker by her bed. 'Here's something, I think. It looks like granola.'

Richard, no longer sleepy, fed her tenderly, spoonful by spoonful. The food gradually made her drowsy. At last she fell asleep. Richard lay on the other bed, restless, turning over, thinking of his parting with Jane the next day, preparing a little speech – something matter-of-fact, almost casual. Something that would let her know, in just a few words, what she had meant to him. No drama.

'How was the night?' Rosemary met Richard in the hall on his way to make a morning cup of coffee. He looked short of sleep. 'Did you get any rest?'

'Not too much, but I'm OK. She talked a lot. She seems more awake at two a.m. than she is all day.'

'It's that way every night. I bet she smoked, too?'

He grimaced. 'Like a chimney. I had to stop her in the end. But we had a good talk.'

Rosemary looked at him sympathetically. 'It must be harder for you, in a way. Jane's always been part of your life, except for the first couple of years before she was born when you were a baby. You won't be able to remember a time when she wasn't part of the world, part of your experience. It isn't quite the same feeling when you gain someone and then lose them again ... We should have come here sooner,' she added. 'It was almost too late. If she'd had the hospice to help before the pain became so bad, she'd have been saved all the anguish and disorientation caused by the move.'

'Nobody expected she'd go down so quickly. I don't think we can blame ourselves.'

A long, luxurious bath helped Richard to recover. By the time he was making his way back to Jane's room, the day nurses had heard all about his interrupted sleep from the night shift.

'You ought to go and have a lie-down in the visitors' room,' Patricia said as Richard was passing the nurses' desk. But what he needed more than a rest was a friendly talk, and he had always found Patricia sympathetic. He knew Jane had made it up with her, but he wasn't so sure about his father. 'It's Dad who finds it hardest,' he said.

'You know, after what he went through in the war – there was death all around him then. This must bring it all back.' As he talked, he became more emotionally involved in his father's past, which had now merged into his own present so that he could have been talking about his own feelings.

Elizabeth, who had come to the desk to pick up some notes, stayed on to listen. She saw he was in a bad way. Something in Richard's story moved her deeply – not what he had been saying about his parents, but what emerged from it of his own feelings, a brother's lament for his sister. She had caught the quaver in his voice, and her own voice broke as she spoke. 'A good cry would do us all good.'

It was what Richard needed. He had been trying to control himself but now, with a great sense of relief, he felt the tears streaming down his cheeks. He realised that he had wanted to cry for a long time. In America he would have done so easily, in similar circumstances; he found it possible to shed his inhibitions there. But in England the old restraint on public display of emotions had reasserted itself. It took Elizabeth's discernment and sympathy to trigger the tears.

Patricia wiped her face and said, 'You must tell us what we can do to help your parents when you've gone.'

'Don't indulge them too much, it wouldn't be good for them. Don't let them stay with Jane all the time.' Richard was back in control now. 'They ought to get away. You should feel free to chase them out occasionally.'

'They're very anxious to be with her. They want to look after her themselves. It's quite natural, but it does mean we're not getting to know Jane so well. Patients talk more freely when they're on their own. It's easier for us to help them when we can know them really well. But, of course, it's lovely for Jane to have her family here.'

'Isn't it harder for you when the patients die if you're close to them?' Richard asked.

'It is, but it's also one of the things that helps us go on. You can do more for a patient if you get to love them, and for that, you have to know them. I don't believe in abstract love, I'm not religious.'

'But aren't most of the staff here religious?' He had

wondered how the nurses found it possible to cope with such a demanding job.

'Yes,' she replied, 'most of them are, very religious indeed.' Patricia knew of Jane's atheism and her family's uneasiness about it. 'David is very religious, too, and some of us were quite concerned when he came. We thought it might make it more difficult for the patients who weren't believers, and for us, too. But it's worked out all right.'

'I can see, though, how real believers might give themselves to this job completely,' Richard said. 'My father was saying that to do this work you must be committed to something, you need tremendous strength to face death day after day. Where can you get it if not outside yourself?'

Patricia bristled slightly but noticeably. 'You don't have to be religious to do this job,' she said firmly. 'But you do have to get something out of it, yes. And I get a lot. It makes me really happy to help the patients, to make them comfortable and peaceful. You know, when I look at someone who comes here suffering pain and misery, and then I watch them falling asleep contented and relaxed . . . that's what I love to see, to know I helped them get this sleep. It makes it all worthwhile.'

Richard was not completely convinced. 'It must be hard here, though, with so many deaths. You must get discouraged, surely?'

'It can be hard, and there are those who can't take it; they don't last more than a few months. Some people are drawn to a hospice because they like to see themselves as angels of mercy. Others have problems of their own – personal or psychological – and they seem to think that working in a hospice, where other people's difficulties are so much greater, will somehow help them solve their own. It doesn't work that way. It's very hard work – physically, emotionally – and you have to be very tough.'

'But you must still get discouraged, however tough you are. How can you put up with it, week after week?'

'When you've helped someone die, peacefully and easily,' Patricia said gently, 'there is nothing better that you can do for another human being, nothing more important or rewarding. If there are several deaths in one week, that makes you very sad. Of course it does. But it also means that several people have gone out of this life without the anguish, without the torment that people usually expect, and you know that in some small way you've helped to bring this about. So one thing balances another. The fact is, I love every minute of it. I am making no self-sacrifice here. I'm getting more, far more, than I'm giving.' She added quietly, 'You can give more to a patient you love. If they've talked to you freely about themselves, about their families, about their pain and happiness in the past, then you've made a friend, a real friend, and how many real friends does one normally make in a lifetime? People who know they're dying don't hold back, usually. They're trusting, open, loving, and then they're so grateful, just like Jane, they keep telling you all the time. It's quite embarrassing,' she finished with a smile.

'I think I understand. But do you always succeed in helping a patient to die peacefully and easily?'

'More often than not, far more often. You see, it's not just love that does it – that's very important, of course, we certainly couldn't succeed without it – but love's been around quite a time. You were talking about religion. Well, there have been all these religious orders for centuries, and they've certainly helped people, even though they had little but love to give. We've got more than that. We can do something to ease the pain, or even stop it, and we can help their relatives as well, if only by talking to them.'

'I don't think I ever talked to a nurse when Jane was in hospital for more than a tenth of the time we've just spent,' Richard said vehemently. 'It's something we feel quite bitter about.'

'Well, you shouldn't. They work those hospital nurses off their feet. Sometimes they don't even have enough time to look after their patients properly. But we are taught that it can often be far more important to talk to a patient or to a member of the family than to do anything else. And we sometimes stay on for an hour or more after a shift is finished to do so. Which is what I'm doing now.' Patricia grinned at him cheerfully.

Victor wanted to be there when Richard said goodbye to Jane. He had accepted that his son was right about leaving, and told him so. The important thing, as David had said, was that the shock of parting might help Jane to let go. He was sorry if he'd made it seem that Richard's decision was selfish. To stay on would have been easy. It needed far more courage and strength of mind to make the decision to go. It needed love.

'You're making too much of it, Dad,' Richard replied uneasily.

'No, Richard. We don't always understand even our own motives, or admit them to ourselves. This is something only you can give her. We couldn't. We have to stay.'

They left it at that. When they went in with Arloc to join Rosemary in Jane's room, the whole family was together again for the first time in several days. Jane communicated her sense of peace to us, and this made the prospect of Richard's departure easier.

Victor had told Adela we would be needing her help. How, he asked her, does one cope with the kind of parting we now had to prepare for? His old fears were surfacing, but she was able to reassure him. She had witnessed many such scenes. How it went would depend to a large extent on them, she said, not on Jane, who had seemed to her quite reconciled. If they made a big thing of it, that could be quite upsetting for Jane. For some patients and families, farewells could be very important. It was a time to bring out thoughts that had been left unsaid, or they might remain locked up forever. People often regretted, for years afterwards, that they had not spoken of the one thing that was on their minds. As far as she could gather, there was nothing like that between Richard and Jane; but one could never be sure. Did he know of anything, she asked Victor, that they needed to say to each other?

No, he said, that wasn't the problem. But Jane was going to be deeply distressed at the parting.

'Would you like me to stand by when Richard leaves? Maybe I can help just by being there?'

'Oh, would you, Adela? I am sure that would help.'

It was what he had been asking for all along, he realised.

Here was someone who was ready to take the burden off them. Jane's friendship with Adela made her almost a member of the family. So far as Jane's dying was concerned, Adela probably understood her better than he did. They had certainly talked about it more directly, more intimately, than he and Jane.

It was almost time to say goodbye. We had discussed taking a family photograph, and Jane who had never liked to have her picture taken, this time agreed quite readily. To Victor, it seemed yet another painful symbol of the leave-taking and the finality of the occasion, but Jane's acquiescence made it unnecessary for him to object.

Arloc first took a picture of Jane while they waited for a nurse to photograph the whole family. Jane was smiling, a small smile, but a real one. It was in her eyes as well as on her lips. The poignancy of the moment differed from the sharp pain Victor had expected. We stood back from the bed and Jane was on her own, as she would be, he thought, when she was dying. She was alone, but she was still smiling as Arloc clicked the shutter.

The family photograph proved more difficult. Rosemary raised Jane up in bed to get her into the group. Jane winced, and the smile disappeared. Now there was an expression of pain on her face which she tried to control with an obvious effort. Elizabeth clicked the shutter quickly before they had all moved into position, and Rosemary lowered Jane back into the pillow, her eyes shut.

The moment had come.

They all went out of the room, leaving Richard alone with his sister. The speech he had prepared had dwindled to a few simple words.

It was Jane who took the initiative. Perhaps she wanted to get it over with.

'You're going now, aren't you, Rich?' she said evenly.

'Yes, Jane, it's time.'

'You've been a good brother to me, Rich,' she went on.

It was Richard who found himself on the verge of tears. 'And you've been a good sister to me,' he said quickly, desperately, as he kissed her lips and almost ran out of the room.

Adela, on the outside, held the door open for him and hurried to the head of Jane's bed. Jane's seeming calm, her even tone, had collapsed in an instant.

'Oh, Adela,' Jane implored her, 'stay with me!' She murmured through her tears: 'I want to sit on your lap, Adela.' At last she could let go, losing the iron control she had imposed for Richard's sake.

Adela hesitated. She couldn't lift Jane off the bed by herself, and this wasn't a good time to ask someone else to help.

Suddenly Jane gave a great sob, and with a huge effort, without waiting for Adela's help, she heaved herself up, turned her body, and pulled herself over towards Adela until she half-sat, half-lay, in her lap. In the past few days Jane had only been able to move her arms and head slightly and very slowly.

We had been watching anxiously through the little window, and thought that now was the time to go in.

Jane looked up as we entered and quickly buried her face in Adela's lap, as if she didn't want to see us. Adela motioned us out of the room urgently, with a single wave of her hand, and yet she managed to do it without appearing too imperious.

Jane's weeping changed to a whimper, like a child's. 'Oh, Adela, he's gone, he's gone.'

Adela's arms went round her, soothing her, stroking her hair, as she continued to cry bitterly for a long time. The weak body, shaking with sobs, was held upright by Adela's strong arms. At last her sobbing eased, then stopped altogether.

Adela beckoned us back into the room. She had wiped Jane's tears away and combed her hair. The hospice routine took over. Jane was as calm and collected as if nothing had happened. She didn't speak of Richard's departure. But she was in pain, and asked for an injection.

She wasn't due for one, yet Elizabeth gave it to her without hesitation. She had been standing by in case Richard's departure produced a crisis. The staff knew what was happening. They had talked about it during the daily report meeting at noon and were on the alert. As soon as Jane had composed herself, word was passed to David Murray and he went in to see if she needed help. When he came out of her room, he told us, 'She's concerned that the process of dying might prove to be a prolonged business.'

It was something that had worried her before, but never as forcefully as now. Richard's departure appeared to mark the end of one stage and the beginning of another. She wasn't quite ready to go yet. She had wanted to live long enough, she told Adela, to say goodbye to Richard and to her friends. Now Richard had gone, and her friends were coming to see her tomorrow. 'When I've seen them all, when I know that my parents are all right, that Dad really can take it, then I'll be ready to go.' She didn't want just to lie there helpless, to get thinner and thinner, looking like a skeleton.

'There is that African tribe I read about,' she said. 'Or is it Indian? Once they decide that the time has come, they just go off into the jungle and settle down to die.'

It was clear that Jane wanted to go, and Victor was ready to acquiesce. He decided it was his duty to help her. Once again he was thinking of euthanasia. If the hospice staff were as open and understanding about dying as they claimed, now was the time for them to show it. He went in search of someone to speak to, and the first person he found was Julia, at the nurses' desk.

The kind of aid he sought would amount, as the law stood, to murder. He tried to sound her out in a roundabout way. Did any of the patients ever ask to be helped out of a life that had become a burden to them? Or did any relatives raise the subject? She listened to him patiently, sympathetically, well aware what was in his mind.

'There was a teenager last month,' she said. 'He told me he couldn't bear to watch his father, and the rest of his family, suffer so much. He thought his father should be helped to die. I asked him: "If I gave you a syringe, would you do it?" '

Victor did not answer, but although she had brought home to him the reality of what he was asking, she had not diverted him from his purpose. She had only shown him that he could not do it himself. But if it was what Jane wanted it should be done. He went to look for David Murray.

'You said that Richard's departure might help her to let go,' Victor said accusingly. 'Well, look what it did to her. I've never seen her so upset. I was afraid this would happen.'

David's attempts to pacify him had little effect. He refused to accept the assurance that Jane's breakdown over Richard was unlikely to recur. He felt she had finally been faced with death as a practical, impending event rather than as a distant, theoretical possibility, and the mental distress was too much for her to bear.

'Why should she go on suffering?' Victor asked. 'You've said yourself it can't be much longer. I know that doctors who really care for their patients, who respect their wishes, will allow them to die when they're ready, even help them if necessary. Hasn't the time come to help Jane?'

'I think I understand how you feel,' David said slowly, 'and I sympathise. I assure you we'll do all we can to minimise Jane's suffering, we'll do nothing to prolong the distress of dying. Certainly, I regard it as part of the doctor's duty to relieve mental distress.' David hesitated, and Victor wondered whether he was looking for a way to agree without admitting it openly so he wouldn't be legally liable.

'To deal with mental distress,' David continued, 'as well as physical distress, it is sometimes necessary to render the patient unconscious. This is part and parcel of traditional medical practice. This we can do, and if it becomes necessary in Jane's case, we will.'

David had conveyed that they would go so far, and no further. He was rejecting Victor's request, gently, expressing his understanding but defining the limits of what was possible and proper in the hospice context. Victor didn't feel that David had refused to help Jane. He was reassured that she wouldn't suffer unnecessarily, that everything would be done to prevent this, and he began to realise that euthanasia was quite inappropriate.

During the night, when she was again wide awake and eager for conversation, Victor reminded Jane of her attempts to help him by talking about the past. He assured her he was no longer afraid. 'I think if I had to go now, I would be ready. As you are. I'm not saying I want to go. You don't, and I don't, but I think we can both take it.'

'I've been waiting to hear you say that for a long time, Dad, and I think I believe you.' There was the slightest trace of hesitation in her voice – not doubt, Victor thought, but perhaps an invitation to produce evidence. He remembered how he had once told Jane he'd accepted her dying, and how she had made him admit that he had not. This time there was no need to lie to her.

'It wasn't just that you helped me to bring it out into the open, Jane. That was only the Jewish part of it; but it isn't only Jews who are afraid to die. There's something more important than that.'

It was being with her, watching her, suffering with her – he had been sharing her dying, as Rosemary and Richard had. They hadn't suffered the actual physical pain she had been experiencing, but they had imagined it often enough. She had told them in Dairy Cottage, before the pain came back, that she was happy in spite of the prognosis Dr. Sullivan had given her. The easy calm that emanated from her at the time, the serenity she radiated when her friends came to see her, the tranquillity she communicated to them, had begun to rub off on him. But, he told her now, he had barely started to come to terms with her dying when the last great rush of pain seemed to be crushing all life out of her, and if it hadn't been for their decision to bring her to the hospice, that unbearable pain would have gone on increasing . . .

He stopped and looked at her quickly, afraid of what he had done. He thought he was telling her how she had helped him to come to terms with death, but in the process he was reminding her of the most painful, most hopeless part of her illness. She lay back now with her eyes half-shut, but she had been listening intently. She understood at once why he had stopped. 'Go on, Dad. I want to hear it. That was one of the times I thought I was dying. I knew that pain could never get better. It was bound to get worse and worse and worse. And that's how it could have ended . . .'

'It could have,' he completed the sentence for her, 'if we hadn't brought you here.'

'Then we would never have had our talk about what the war did to you.'

'And I suppose you would never have known that you helped me to get rid of my fear?'

'Dad,' she spoke firmly now, 'you're up to your tricks again. You're trying to make me think it's all my doing, to make me feel good. But it's the hospice that did it, not me. I tried to get through to you at Dairy Cottage, and failed. But here it worked. I told the nurses I was worried about you. And they kept saying, "Talk to him about it".'

'Is there anything else you want, Jane? Anything at all?'

'Yes,' she said. 'Kiss me.'

Victor was not a demonstrative person. He had not often caressed the children, even when they were small. Sometimes he would let them sit on his lap, smooth their hair in a gesture of affection. He wished now he had been less inhibited.

He bent over her and kissed her lips. 'Go to sleep now,' he said quietly as she shut her eyes. He crossed over to the window. It was not as dark as it had been. The silence was broken by a twitter, a muted uncertain noise, as if a bird were slowly coming out of sleep. This call was answered, first by one bird, then by others, all sounding equally sleepy. The exchange soon ended, and silence fell once more – but Jane was not asleep.

A bird began to sing, properly this time. Again others answered, joining in gradually until the singing came from all directions. As more and more joined the chorus the sound grew louder in volume, until the burst of exuberant joy and beauty filled the room. There were many different birds and many varieties of song, yet they all merged into a harmonious whole like a well-trained orchestra. Victor turned his back to the window and looked at Jane.

She was listening intently, her eyes wide open, following him around the room as he walked back to the head of the bed. They waited together as the music rose to an exultant crescendo and then suddenly fell away except for isolated notes. It was hard to believe that these musicians worked without a conductor. It was as if they sang with great joy to be alive as a new day began.

Jane still waited, alert to the occasional calls which came less and less frequently. Victor was deeply moved. What was she thinking? She looked at him.

'How lovely that was,' he said gently.

'You must have heard the dawn chorus before, Dad?'

'I never listened properly, never heard it until today,' he answered. 'How quiet it is now.'

The sky was a soft, misty grey.

'They'll be singing again soon,' she said, 'when the sun comes up – but not like that. You ought to listen more, Dad, and to look around you, not spend all the time among your books and papers. The world is very beautiful . . .'

A moment later she was asleep.

Chapter 15

When Jane woke up on Wednesday she experienced the pain of parting all over again. Her lips moved slowly after Rosemary asked her if she'd slept well. Her 'Yes' sounded uncertain.

'Where's Richard?' she asked. 'Is he coming today?'

Her mother said gently, 'No, darling. You'll remember in a minute. He's left with Arloc. They're on their way to America. Richard rang up from the airport to send you his love – and Arloc too.' Jane still looked puzzled, so Rosemary went on: 'Remember, they said goodbye to you last night?'

Then Jane remembered. 'He's really gone,' she wailed. 'I shan't see him again.' She turned her head to hide her tears and cried quietly to herself. Rosemary stroked her hair and tried to convey that she understood how terrible this loss, this final parting, was. She could only remind Jane how much Richard had loved her, how Arloc had grown to love and understand her.

'I want to die quickly,' she said. 'I wonder if I'll die soon. I want it to be over with.'

'I'm sure it won't be long. Perhaps Richard and Arloc not being here will make it easier for you to go . . . You may feel, deep down, that you don't have to stay any more now. It was hard for Richard to leave you, you must know that, because it's so hard for you.' Rosemary lit a cigarette for Jane. 'We're going to find it terribly difficult to get used to being without you. But, Jane, you'll always be around for us. We have so many ways to remember you.'

She grew calmer at last. She lay looking out of the window

at the sky. The morning was grey and cool, as summer mornings often are in England. The clouds merged into a continuous cover, cutting off the sun and giving no hint that soon they would disperse to allow the light through.

Once again the hospice life reached out to Jane. Julia asked if she would like a visit from Bunty, her little dog. Jane had had no thought of ever touching an animal again and was delighted at the suggestion. When Julia brought Bunty, a griffin, into her room, she asked, 'Would you like her on your bed, Jane? She'll wriggle about, you must tell me if it bothers you.'

Jane wasn't bothered. Bunty joined her on the bed, and Jane smiled with happiness as the dog licked her face and fingers, nuzzling against her, bursting with love. Julia stood watching in case Bunty's enthusiasm got out of hand.

Rosemary remembered the day when her own mother had died, quite unexpectedly. Rosemary had found her in the morning, arms resting over the bedcover, the telephone within easy reach. Only the colour of her face and the dropped line of her jaw indicated that she wasn't asleep. Even the cold touch of her flesh didn't convince Rosemary that her mother had died. Rosemary had been on holiday and it seemed terrible not to have said goodbye. In great distress she knocked at the house next door. The dog, which was always gentle and friendly, that day leaped out in apparent rage and fury and had to be restrained from attacking Rosemary. Perhaps it had picked up a sense or a smell of fear, of stress – or of death? Animals are often thought to be especially sensitive to these situations, but certainly Bunty showed no such reaction. Jane's death was drawing very close, but she wasn't afraid. Bunty wriggled about on Jane's bed, licking the feeble fingers that tried to stroke her.

Later that morning Jane asked for another injection. For the first time since her arrival in the hospice, help took some time coming. She lay with her eyes closed, but finally asked: 'Could you see where they've got to? I really need that injection.'

Rosemary went to find help. Elizabeth was at the nurses' desk. Her usual ready smile vanished when she saw Rosemary.

'How awful! I'll come right away. I forgot all about it. How could I . . .?'

She hurried to Jane's room with a syringe and long apologies. As she gave the injection, her movements were quicker than usual, but still gentle. 'There now, did you feel that?'

'Not a bit. But I'm not comfortable . . .'

'You've slipped down in the bed. If your mother takes the other side of the sheet, we'll pull it right up and needn't move your body.' She grasped one side of the sheet and Rosemary took the other. 'One. two, three, *hup* . . .' Quickly and easily Jane was lifted higher in the bed. 'Did that hurt?'

'No. That's much better, thanks. I'm sorry I bothered you, but I really needed that injection.' Jane was already beginning to relax. 'I'm sure you're very busy.'

'No,' Elizabeth said bluntly, 'it wasn't that. I just forgot. Wasn't that terrible of me?'

Jane smiled back at Elizabeth's disarming candour. Rosemary admired the nurse's courage for telling the truth so easily, and felt no anxiety that such an oversight would happen again. Soon the injection worked and, with her pain eased, Jane was once more peaceful and contented.

David Murray arrived for his morning visit and talked to us after he had spent some time with Jane. He was his usual calm self. Today Victor was calmer, too. He had been acting as if he'd been wound up so tightly that he could only function at speed. Now his sense of urgency and stress had eased; he no longer moved and spoke as if barely containing an enormous tension. But he was unable to relax for long. Rosemary realised that his nature was such that he couldn't just wait for the inevitable. He had to keep on struggling and fighting towards the goal of a peaceful death for Jane. She knew that at this time he must pursue an active role, whereas she could only wait.

David gave us fresh news of her physical condition. 'The tumour in her abdomen has blocked off her system,' he said. 'We've had no results from our efforts at clearing her bowels. This points to a complete stoppage.'

'In that case,' Rosemary asked, 'does she need to eat? It's a tremendous effort, but she feels she has a duty to take nourishment. If her system isn't absorbing anything, must she really go on eating?'

'Absolutely not,' David said firmly. 'Some patients have their meals right up to the end, but only if they want to.'

'She'll be glad.'

'Patients sometimes eat to please the people looking after them. It's their way of returning an expression of love – by accepting the gift of food.'

'Oh, she hates eating now.' Rosemary found it easy to talk to David. 'Jane seems to think she may die very soon now.'

'It's possible. There are those who can put into operation a kind of primitive mechanism that early man possessed, and most of us have lost – an ability to switch off, you might say. She may well be able to decide that this is the time . . .' He was quiet for a moment, then went on, 'Sometimes it's necessary for a doctor to give permission, as it were, for a patient to die. This sounds a bit like playing God' – he smiled apologetically – 'but a patient can feel a responsibility towards the doctor, a duty to respond to care and attention by going on living and thereby showing she appreciates it. Then the dying person needs to be gently nudged into realising that this is no longer necessary. The doctor has to see the facts as they are, the biological facts. It's also the doctor's responsibility to allow the scales to tip toward death in certain situations. When I talk about "permission to die," that's what I mean. It's a matter of tipping the scales.' He paused again. 'This probably sounds very arrogant,' he said quietly.

'Isn't it more arrogant to refuse to accept death?' Rosemary asked.

'You may be right.'

Jane's world had shrunk to her bed now. Her only remaining possessions were a favourite ashtray, a stoneware vase made by her mother, her shawls and her toilet bag. But her personality was intact, her identity hadn't been drowned in drugs or crushed by pain. Nor did she feel a need to hide herself away. Her life was real, and she continued to take great pleasure in communicating with the people who came to her room to look after her, or just to talk. She was still enjoying new experiences, listening with interest to whatever her visitors had to say.

One of the volunteers kept Jane company while Victor and Rosemary had lunch together. When Julia introduced her, Rosemary could only think, How young this girl is. She can't be more than seventeen. How can she possibly know what to say to someone mortally ill?

The girl smiled happily and sat down by Jane's bed. She began to talk freely and enthusiastically as one healthy person talks to another, and Jane responded easily. If she felt resentment or envy at her visitor's vitality, she gave no sign. 'We had a good talk,' she said to us, when we got back.

That afternoon Jane told Dorothy and Julia that she was happier than she'd ever been. 'The world is such a beautiful place. I know that now, I never really saw it before. I think I'm so lucky to be here, in the best place in such a lovely world.' She told them there was nothing more important in life than being born and dying. 'At birth,' she said, 'I knew nothing. At death, I know everything that I will ever know, and everything around me is good, not evil. That's a good way to die.'

They were making her comfortable in bed, having just turned her over. 'You're so good to me,' Jane went on. 'Everyone makes such a fuss of me . . .' She broke off and laughed. 'I'm beginning to sound like a stuck record, going on and on. You'll get sick of the sound.'

'We won't get sick of it, Jane,' Julia assured her. 'It's good to hear you say these things. We enjoy looking after you.'

Dorothy smiled her agreement. 'You really do have remarkable control over your legs, Jane, even though you can't move them properly. It's very noticeable when we change your position.'

'I used to do a lot of yoga before I got ill. It was very relaxing, especially when I couldn't sleep. There's only one thing that worries me. I wish I knew what it was going to be like – dying, I mean. I'm a bit scared of that, but I suppose nobody knows . . .'

Julia looked at her gravely. 'I think I can tell you,' she said. 'You'll just go to sleep and slip away without even waking up.' She spoke quietly, but with assurance.

There was a moment's silence while Jane absorbed this. 'That sounds good to me.'

Julia went on: 'I've watched a lot of people while they died, and that's what will most probably happen to you.'

Jane was content. Now, free of the constraints of the future, free of possible disciplines that she would resent and probable defeats that might crush her, she had only to deal with the present, and it was manageable, limited, under control. She seemed to have no fear left in her.

That afternoon, hot and mellow with sunshine, a group of Jane's friends came down from London, bringing strawberries, melon and mangos for her, not knowing that she wasn't eating any longer. It wasn't long before they realised that this was their last meeting. Kate, the first to go in, saw at once how much weaker Jane had become since she visited her on Sunday, three days ago. Jane's eyes were too weak to see her clearly, but she recognised the voice. Kate hugged and kissed her. Jane asked, 'Tell me what you're wearing today. You always wear such nice things. Describe what you look like.'

'Oh, I haven't got dressed up for you today.' Kate tried to paint a word picture. 'I put on my Indian skirt – the browney one with the figures on it, remember? Then I've got a white shirt and some beads – the wooden ones – round my neck. That's about it. Oh, yes, I found it too hot to wear the boots that go well with this skirt, so I put on sandals instead.'

'Now I know how you look.' Jane spoke with contentment. 'It is a lovely day, isn't it? I can feel the sun in the air.'

There was no hint of envy in her voice, Kate thought, remembering how Jane had always loved the sun. She tried to keep her own voice light and cheerful as she asked: 'Still glad you came here, then?' When Jane smiled and nodded, Kate added: 'You do look lovely, you know. Really happy.'

They were silent together. Aware of her friend's weakness and anxious not to tire her, Kate waited for Jane to speak. Her next words were full of pleasure at the smell of the freesias Kate had brought. 'What a beautiful world it is!' she added. 'We really should always enjoy it, every moment.' She gave Kate a last message for Michael.

Jane's other two friends waited outside on the sunny

terrace for their turn to see her. From a distance it might have been a holiday scene: the group of young people sitting chatting under a sunshade, looking out over the open countryside beyond the garden. But as they each went in to her it was increasingly obvious to them that Jane had not much longer to live. She was failing rapidly; her body was very frail, she was almost blind, her voice was sometimes merely a whisper. Only her happiness remained, and the sense of peace that surrounded her, which seemed to intensify, not diminish, as the day went on.

When she talked with her friends – quietly, a few words at a time – she was working hard to help them accept that she was dying. If she could show them it was possible to die in peace when their time came, that would be a great thing to leave behind her. And in the act of accepting the gift, they would be returning it to her and making her own dying easier. She was ready to say goodbye.

We took turns to make sure Jane wasn't getting too tired. Although she didn't like to say so herself, it was obvious that she needed a rest after only a brief talk. One of us would stay with her while she dozed, then another friend would go in. When Linda, Jane's childhood friend, emerged, she was bewildered and weeping. 'I can't believe it,' she cried. 'I just can't believe it.' Linda had visited Jane every few days since her return to England from Greece. She had followed the progress of the illness and knew what had been happening – at least, as much as the family had known. But it was still hard for her to accept that there was now no hope of remission, no chance at all. She wept, struggling with this knowledge, and the rest of the group under the sunshade tried to comfort her.

Jane had noticed Linda's distress. 'Don't let Linda go home alone,' she said to her mother. 'She shouldn't drive on her own.' That moved Linda even more. 'That she should be thinking of me at a time like this,' she said, and broke down again.

In the evening Jane seemed completely at peace. The pain of Richard's departure was apparently gone – she had forgotten it, or perhaps accepted it. She had said goodbye to him and to the friends she cared most for, and she made her decision. 'I am ready,' she said. 'I want it to be tonight.'

She lay with her face towards the glow of the evening sky that came through the window. The sun had set some time before but there was still plenty of light.

It was one of those times when the world seemed full of meaning to Rosemary. If only one could find the secret, everything would fall into place. She felt that even life and death might cease to be a mystery and their meaning become easy to understand – the explanation was very close. All the sights and sounds of this June evening should form a complete whole: the nightingales singing the lovely song that is really their battle cry, the sliver of moon in the glowing sky, her dying daughter on the bed – these were all parts of the pattern, if only she could see it clearly. Perhaps Jane's new-found tranquillity and happiness were signs that the mystery had been solved for her.

Among Jane's papers we found a poem she had written in hospital:

> I try to fill my head with stars,
> To drift in space
> And find peace.
>
> But tonight
> The stars are far away,
> Peace will not come.

Now at last she was at peace.

Rosemary tried to describe to her the beauty of the evening, the light in the sky, the patches of deeper darkness under the hedge. Then she saw a movement. 'There's a rabbit, Jane. He's just come through the hedge. He's eating the grass on the other side of the road . . .'

'A rabbit!' Jane was thrilled. 'I must see him. Lift me up, quick!'

'It will hurt you.' Rosemary said doubtfully.

'Oh, Mum,' Jane begged, 'my last rabbit!'

Then Rosemary knew she must help her do whatever she wanted, even though she couldn't see clearly. She put her arms under Jane's shoulders and raised the weak body up in bed. Jane peered over in the direction of the hedge.

She couldn't see anything. The world was a blur.

'He's gone, Jane. He must have heard my voice. But he was there,' she said firmly. 'A lovely young rabbit. Perhaps if we keep quiet, he'll come out again.'

Back in bed Jane lay with her face still turned to the open window, waiting for the rabbit. The light was hazy as the dusk deepened, and the air that came through the window smelled of the day's sunlight. Soon it grew dark. The rabbit had not reappeared, but Jane did not complain. Her memory of other rabbits had been refreshed by this last visitor.

Victor came into the room looking worried. 'Jane,' he said hesitantly, 'Michael has just called, he wants to come and talk to you.'

'No.' Her reaction was immediate. 'I'm too tired.' She lay deep in the bed, her voice strained. 'I don't want to see him.'

'You've been saying you wanted to sort out any past mis-understandings with your friends and set things straight. You owe it to him to talk things through.'

'I'm too tired,' Jane snapped back. 'I've told Kate what to say to him.'

'Jane.' Victor would not accept her refusal. 'You really ought . . .'

Rosemary cut in, 'Why don't you talk on the telephone? You could have a long rest first and speak to him later.'

Jane considered this in silence for a moment. 'I know,' said Victor, 'a Zorza solution for you, Jane. Let's toss a coin.'

She began to come round slightly. 'You know perfectly well we always do the opposite of what the coin says – even if we do remember which side meant what . . . Oh, all right then. If you must.'

'So it's heads you'll speak to him . . .'

'Does it matter?' she asked. But she added grudgingly, 'Heads, then.'

The coin came down heads. She wavered and began to give in. 'Well, I suppose if I smoked all the time I could manage. But I'll have to be alone,' she said emphatically. 'I don't want anyone here while I talk to him.'

'Darling, you can't be alone if you smoke,' Rosemary objected. 'You might burn the whole place down if the cigarette slips.'

'I can't have anyone listening. I won't do it then, not if someone's got to sit and watch me.'

'Suppose I put in ear plugs and promise not to look at your face, only the cigarette. How about that?'

So it was agreed. The telephone was brought into her room and plugged in. Victor went off to call Michael. When he didn't return, Rosemary went to investigate and found him in a state of confusion, half laughing, half in anguish. 'You'd better come with me,' he whispered, 'I don't think I can face this alone.' Mystified, Rosemary followed him back into the room.

'Jane, I'm afraid I was too late to stop Michael. By the time I got through, he'd left. He's on his way.'

Jane, who had recovered from her earlier anger, now exploded in a surprisingly strong new burst. 'What a shit thing to do! How could he do this to me? Just like him. What a a swine he is!'

'He was on his way to the station when I called. There's no way to stop him. He'll get here about one in the morning, I suppose.'

'I won't see him!' Victor lit a cigarette for her, and she puffed hard at it, her eyes full of tears. 'I was expecting to die tonight. Now I can't die if he's to come here.'

'Jane,' Victor remonstrated, 'he can't stop you dying if it's time for you to go. When your body is ready, you'll die. You don't have to see him if you don't want to.'

'You don't understand. I'll have to if he comes all this way.' Her face was still distorted with misery and rage. 'I'm too tired to see him,' she repeated. 'I won't see him.'

The cigarette slipped from her agitated fingers and the hot ash fell on her hands. 'Now I've burned myself! It hurts terribly,' she said accusingly. Her limps fingers fumbled together, attempting to rub the injured part but lacking the strength even to locate the burn. Feverishly, Rosemary rubbed cream into her hands, trying to see the burn, to calm and reassure her.

She was acting like a spoiled brat, we both thought, and then felt ashamed of the thought. A moment ago we had been ready for a solemn, quiet ending. Jane was going to put her head on the pillow, shut her eyes, and drift off to sleep easily, comfortably, just as she wanted it, just as she had been promised would happen. Now this peaceful ending was threatened. The whole thing was degenerating into farce, Victor thought angrily. We reminded her that she always felt like talking in the middle of the night. She could sleep now, then talk later.

'I shan't sleep,' she said defiantly. 'How can I sleep after this? My finger hurts too much.'

Rosemary's patience was slipping away. 'Of course you'll sleep.' For the first time since Jane's illness, she spoke as to a little girl, rather an unreasonable and naughty little girl at that. 'You've slept well every night here. You'll have your usual injection, more if you need it.'

'Well, give me another cigarette, then.'

'No!' We both shouted together. 'No more cigarettes!'

Meanwhile, Elizabeth had told David Murray that Jane's calm, steady journey towards death had been unexpectedly interrupted. He came in, allowing us to escape and find time to pull ourselves together. We went to the kitchen to make some tea.

Victor was appalled at the collapse of calm and order. 'This is terrible,' he kept saying, 'terrible.' When David joined them, having succeeded in settling Jane down, Victor said, 'It's all coming apart. What are we to do?'

But David remained unruffled. 'Once the pattern has been set, then it will be maintained,' he said. 'Unexpected things do happen, there may be upsets ... But things will right themselves, get back on course. You'll see that basically nothing has changed.'

Rosemary was less upset by the incident; indeed, she was almost glad it had happened. The turmoil and stress of life were still affecting Jane. 'I feel a sense of relief,' she admitted. 'This evening had begun to seem like a scene from a Victorian novel – the lovely girl on the bed, the moon, the nightingales. It was too good to be true. This is the real Jane!'

'I know what you mean.' David smiled in sympathy. 'But before this happened, had you felt she was losing her identity because of the drugs? Were you worrying that she was becoming a zombie? Or have you thought all along that she was the same Jane?'

'Oh, yes, definitely the same Jane. She's been happy and content, but you couldn't call it a personality change or anything like that. And she's certainly not become a zombie. Things just went wrong this evening. It's an emotional business for her.'

Rosemary settled down for the night beside Jane, still stoutly maintaining that she wouldn't doze off. But she slept soundly through the night. Even the arrival of the night nurses with their whispered warning, 'Your injection, Jane,' failed to wake her.

She didn't hear Michael's taxi driving past her window to the front door of the hospice.

Michael had decided to come to the hospice when Kate got back from seeing Jane, he told us later. As soon as he heard that Jane hadn't much longer to live, he knew he must go to her again. 'Maybe dashing off to see her now fits in with the way we were,' he told Kate, 'always rushing here and there to meet each other – driving, travelling . . .'

Even Victor's misgivings, clearly evident when Michael phoned the hospice, hadn't discouraged him. 'Victor and Rosemary will need support tonight, maybe I can give it to them.' In any case, he had to go. And later, when we talked about the events of that night, he told us: 'It's not really the thing to do to intrude on a family matter, but that's the way Jane and I were . . . untidy . . . We missed too many chances together. I wasn't going to miss this one.'

Michael remembered that journey vividly. He had never before travelled in a train where he could sit looking out of the back window of the carriage. He watched patterns of light forming shapes of colour and movement that increased his sense of unreality. The strangeness of the journey served to underline the fact that his long relationship with Jane was coming to an end.

He wondered whether he would make it in time. Would she be able to see him? Would she *want* to see him? Or was she still upset and bitter, as Kate had told him, that he hadn't come to visit her alone for several weeks, that there was always somebody with him? It was too late to try to sort out his reasons for bringing Ruth along on these occasions; they were too complicated.

The memory of his first painful breakup with Jane returned, but he tried to forget it. It had been a damaging experience and the present was hard enough to deal with, without the pain of old wounds. They'd worked out all their bad feelings about each other even before cancer struck Jane – they'd settled their old accounts. At least, that's what he'd thought until he talked to Kate. She gave him the impression that Jane was still angry with him. And his talk on the phone with Victor confirmed it.

When the taxi dropped him at the door of the hospice, he hesitated, reluctant to ring the bell and wake the whole place. To his surprise, a nurse was waiting by the door to let him in. 'We heard the taxi coming,' she explained, and went on to say that Jane was asleep, but her father was expecting him. She led him in.

'I didn't want to upset you,' Michael began hesitantly.

Victor explained that he was only concerned that the rhythm of Jane's dying shouldn't be disturbed. It was important she should put her affairs in order. But she was also exhausted, and in no state to talk any more. 'We were relieved that the decision whether you should come or not was taken from us.' Michael felt even guiltier than before.

When Victor suggested he could ask the nurses to make up a bed for him in the visitors' room, Michael refused at first, but finally consented.

At six o'clock in the morning Victor knocked on the door to tell him that Jane was waking up. He must come immediately, there might be no other chance. Michael went in to see her, but could make no contact. He spoke to her. She stared straight ahead, not recognising him, not answering. He held her hand, but she didn't respond to his touch. Now he could see and believe that Jane was really dying.

It's too late, he thought. *I came too late*. Still, he was glad to be with her. He waited beside her bed in silence until Victor took him to breakfast.

While Adela sat with Jane, she began to come to the surface again. Adela asked, 'Jane, would you like to see Michael? He's been waiting for hours to see you. He's so patient.'

'Has he been here? I can't remember . . .'

'He was here with you earlier, but you weren't really awake.'

'Yes.' Jane's mind was clearing rapidly. 'I'd like him to come. But don't let anyone else in, will you? I must see him alone – it's important.' She was struggling to wake completely, to talk clearly.

The anger had gone. When Michael returned to her bedside, she didn't speak of the resentment she had mentioned to Kate. Instead, she told him she knew how unhappy she had made him when they were lovers. 'I am sorry . . . very sorry.'

They were close to each other again. They said little, but the meaning behind their words was clear to both. He held her hand. Their past differences were forgotten; only the understanding remained.

When the moment of parting came, Jane watched Michael as he moved towards the door. Suddenly she asked: 'Am I dying?' She had been so sure her end was near, he thought, and yet it hadn't come. Now he looked into her large, still luminous eyes and wondered what she meant.

It was too much. He could only stammer a quick 'Yes', and rush from the room.

Adela had kept her eye on the door to make sure no one else walked in while he was with Jane. She knew that Jane would want to see her when Michael had left. She would be upset, but she would prefer to hide it from her parents, as she had done after Richard had gone. Jane had made it clear she hoped to spare them as much distress as possible. 'They deserve to be happy,' she'd said to Adela a few days before. Now Adela went quickly into her room to comfort her. 'I told him how sorry I am,' Jane said.

It took some time before Jane had recovered and could once more present a smiling face to her parents. Victor wanted to be doing things for her, expressing his love by action.

'Would you like some music now?' When she nodded, he put on a tape of one of Mozart's last string quartets, some of the most serene of all classical music. The notes sounded clear, soft and gentle, as if falling on the air.

'How lovely that is,' Jane's voice was as quiet as the music. 'You're making it so beautiful for me to die.'

Rosemary felt that Jane was completely at peace with the world. She seemed to exist in a timeless state. She would doze, sleep, wake – all without any knowledge of the passing of time.

She asked, 'How long do they think I'll live?' and her question was calm, dispassionate, with no hint of fear.

Rosemary answered, 'Even if they knew, I don't think it would mean much to you. You seem to be on a different wavelength where it doesn't matter what time it is, or what day it is. If they said, "Six hours more," then you might sleep for that six hours and not know you'd been asleep.'

'I suppose so,' she agreed sleepily, drifting off again.

It had been some time since Jane had asked for anything other than painkillers, cigarettes, or an occasional sip of apple juice. There seemed to be nothing she felt a need for. But some memory must have stirred, for she asked, her words soft and slow: 'There is one thing . . . I suppose its impossible . . .' The voice came as if she were speaking through a muffling curtain. 'You know how I've always loved velvet? I would like to touch velvet again before I die. I don't suppose it would be possible . . .?'

'Oh yes it will,' Adela answered at once. 'I'll bring you a piece when I get back from lunch.'

Jane was content, but 'after lunch' wasn't soon enough for Victor. She should have what she wanted right away. He left the room and began to ask everyone in sight if there was any velvet in the building. Maybe someone lived close enough to pop out and return with a piece? Or was there a shop nearby? Soon everybody was hunting for velvet. Phone calls were made, trips to the shopping centre, a quick visit to the nurses' living quarters. No hint of the upheaval came back to Jane, but in a short time, there were three pieces of velvet for her to choose from. She smiled with pleasure as Dorothy gave them to her to touch, one by one. She chose the softest, a small oblong of deep pink silk velvet. Dorothy laid it on her shoulder so that she could feel its warm texture against her skin, and there it remained for the rest of her life.

Sue, who had helped Rosemary to find the wild flowers, now brought a fresh rosebud from her garden. She laid it on the pillow beside Jane. 'It looks so good next to your hair. The colour is just right for you,' she said. The rosebud was a deep, rich red.

'I've always wanted to wear a rose in my hair,' Jane murmured, 'but I never quite had the nerve . . .'

Sue carefully pushed the stem of the flower into her hair, behind the ear, making sure there were no thorns to catch her skin.

From that time on, Jane wore a rose in her hair. When the first bloom withered, it was replaced. If the nurses had to turn Jane to keep her circulation going, or to give her an injection or make her comfortable, they always replaced the rose. The piece of velvet and the rose were handled with the greatest gentleness and delicacy, as if nothing in the world was more precious.

Jane spent many hours asleep. When she woke, it was clear her mind was relaxed and untroubled by nightmares. She spoke suddenly: 'Is that you, Mum?'

Rosemary moved closer, bending low over the bed in case Jane could still see something of her face. 'Yes, it's me. Dad'll be back soon.'

'Lie down on the bed beside me.' It was a humble request, not a command.

Rosemary longed to hug Jane, to hold her closely again, but she hesitated. Her body seemed so fragile now, almost soft enough to be damaged by physical contact. 'I don't want to hurt you,' she said.

But she reached up and half-lay, half-leaned against the bed, as close to Jane as she could get. There wasn't room enough for the two of them to lie side by side on the narrow bed.

She put her arms loosely round her daughter's still form. Then Jane moved over her own body slowly and with great difficulty until she lay even closer to Rosemary. With a gesture slow and clumsy, but conveying infinite love, she moved a limp arm round to embrace her mother.

'I do love you, Mum,' she said.

It was a moment to remember – a time when all the minor

233

disagreements of life, the jealousies, the disappointments and stresses were swept away and forgotten.

There had been none of the depth of tension between her and Jane that had existed between Jane and Victor. She had often been in the middle, acting as a buffer, trying to explain one to the other, to bring about mutual understanding. Jane knew Rosemary didn't take sides between her and Victor, so she hadn't resented her as a go-between. She had been close to her mother since the storms of adolescence had died down.

In the late afternoon, Patricia went to see Jane on her way home. 'I just came in before I went off duty. You may not be here on Saturday . . . of course, I'd like you to be, but I know you'll be glad to get it over with . . .' She stumbled slightly, not knowing quite how to put it into words. 'But I did want to say goodbye properly to you.'

Jane had always valued the affection of family and friends, even if she'd sometimes rebelled against the disciplines love imposes. But to be loved by people who had been, only a week before, absolute strangers was a constant source of wonder and happiness. She couldn't thank them enough; she wanted to give presents to express her own love and gratitude. She tried hard to make everyone understand how much it meant to her to be in a place so 'good'.

'Once I'd have found that a trite thing to say,' she said. 'In fact, all the things that have meant most to me these last months would have seemed corny or sentimental before I got ill.'

Her happiness was clearly apparent. She had no guilt about being helpless and dependent on others. She had always loved to give, but she seemed at last to accept that she could now only receive. Perhaps she realised she could only give by taking – with gratitude and without guilt. Her needs were fulfilled without question and without resentment. In return she lavished praise on everyone who served her, and did so with humility. Perhaps it was the first time in her life that she didn't feel she had to live up to someone else's expectations of behaviour or achievement.

Absorbed in the most difficult task of her life, that of dying, she had no doubts left.

Rosemary said to David Murray, 'I know she's not religious, so I hesitate to use the words, but it's almost as if she were in a state of grace.'

'I think you could say that,' David agreed.

We no longer felt sickened by the cigarette smoke. All too soon there would be no more smoke; it seemed impossible that such a little thing could have upset us so much. But as Jane's weakness increased, her smoking became even more perilous. Someone always had to watch the cigarette wobbling insecurely between her limp fingers, holding the ashtray ready to trap the blocks of burned ash. But if the sitter's attention was distracted for a moment, the cigarette might fall, singeing Jane's chest or shoulders. On one occasion it took several minutes to rescue a glowing stub.

Rosemary told David she was afraid they might burn the place down.

'We do have flame-proof sheets,' he said, unworried. 'But if you like, we can have a bucket of sand kept outside the door in case of emergency.'

Victor had another, more serious concern. He spoke to David privately about it. 'What about the death rattle? Isn't that very alarming? I've read about this horrible noise going on and on.' He feared that Jane, perhaps semiconscious in her last moments, might hear her own death rattle and realise what was happening.

'That we can deal with,' David answered. 'The so-called rattle is the result of fluid in the back of the throat causing a bubbling, choking noise. An injection of hyoscene will dry up the secretions if necessary.'

At five o'clock on the day Jane had said goodbye to Michael, David went in to see her. Her periods of waking had been shorter, and further apart. It was many hours since she had last opened her eyes. She lay still, her breathing light but regular. Now she was deeply asleep, perhaps unconscious.

David signalled us to follow him out of the room on to the terrace.

He was clearly moved. 'She's going, isn't she?'

There seemed no doubt of it.

Victor asked unsteadily: 'How long do you think she has?'

'It's hard to say. Perhaps as little as two hours.'

Even now, when Jane gave no sign of hearing what was said, none of the hospice staff ever talked as if she were not in the room. They spoke to her and included her in every conversation. They told us that sick and dying people often hear quite clearly what is being said around them, even though they seem unconscious.

The promise that Jane wouldn't be left alone was easy to keep. Two old friends who had known her since she was a small child, and had opened their home to us all when she came back from Greece, sat with her for long periods. Sometimes we talked, sometimes we sat in silence, not because we felt we shouldn't or couldn't talk, but because silence was more natural than speech. The presence of these friends was a great comfort to us, helping Jane on her last journey. It was a link with all the bedside vigils of past centuries when relatives and friends silently watched and waited. It was a reminder that death was inevitable, a natural part of life's pattern, not an isolated event that was destroying Jane, but a universal experience.

David had warned us that, now her bowels were obstructed, she might start to vomit. This could precipitate her death, but would make it a horrible event.

'We must look out for any signs,' he said. 'Then we'll act to prevent it with injections.'

We watched Jane with this possibility always in our minds. Dr. Brown, who had admitted her to the hospice, was back on duty again. 'She looks so peaceful,' he said; 'we must do our best to keep her this way.' But his words upset Rosemary. *They must succeed in this. There should be no question that Jane must die in peace.* She knew she was being unreasonable, that everything possible would be done. Dr. Brown had not been expressing any doubt, merely reaffirming an intention.

Jane continued to lie still, peaceful.

That night Victor stayed with Jane while Rosemary slept in the visitors' room.

She woke suddenly in the middle of the night without

apparent reason and, without thinking, got out of bed and walked down the corridor towards Jane's room. Outside the night was dark and still; inside, dim lights shone in the nursing station. Both night nurses must be busy.

There was a soft light in the room. Nora and Victor were bending over Jane.

He was surprised to see Rosemary. 'How extraordinary . . . Jane's just this minute woken for the first time. Can you hear what she's trying to say?'

Rosemary bent over her daughter, afraid that the terrible sickness was on its way. 'Darling,' she said. 'Are you all right?'

Jane mumbled something indistinct.

Rosemary spoke more urgently: 'Do you feel sick, Jane?'

Her answer was clearly heard by them all. 'Sick – pain,' she said.

These words were enough, and Nora was ready with the injection. Jane sank once again into a deep sleep.

The next morning her breathing had changed. There was no longer a continuous flow of air in and out of her body; one sharp intake of breath would be followed by a silence lasting several seconds. Then she would exhale in a long sigh. Although the period between inhalation and exhalation varied a few seconds each time, it always seemed interminable. The silence was a vacuum, a foretaste of death.

The nurses came regularly to give injections, to move her, to moisten her mouth. They talked to her even though she was unconscious, explaining what they were doing in low, calm voices. The halting breaths dragged on. But the pulse at her neck beat with surprising vigour.

Previous mornings had been filled with the daily chores of cleaning and tidying. Now these activities had ceased. The water jug had been moved, quietly and without comment, when Jane stopped drinking. Offers of food had ceased when she didn't want to eat any more. The cleanliness of her room was no longer important: dust settled on furniture and floor, and nobody cared. Jane had priority, not the hospice routine.

In the silence, broken only by the murmuring voices of the nurses, it was even more noticeable that the tending of

Jane's body was a form of communication. The moistening of her mouth, the time taken to rub her body with sweet-smelling lotion, emphasised the concern of the hospice staff.

During the day Jane's breathing changed again, growing harsh and thick, wheezing in and out of her throat with apparent difficulty, making us wonder whether this might not be the beginning of the death rattle after all. Her face became red and congested, but her expression remained serene.

'She has pneumonia,' Dr. Brown said. 'This will save her.' What he meant was that pneumonia would help her to die more quickly. He prescribed drugs to clear her congested lungs. The possibility of giving antibiotics to prolong her life was never mentioned. The pulse at her throat still beat strongly. He watched it with compassion. 'That's the penalty of being young. She has a strong body,' he said.

As we came out of Jane's room, Julia asked, 'Perhaps you'd like to be in with Jane? We're just going to turn her. It's possible that the fluid on her lungs will shift when we move her. She may go very suddenly.'

Jane lay as we had left her.

Her body was limp as they raised it in their arms. We watched while they laid her gently down in the bed. The heavy breathing went on; the pulse at her neck beat as strongly as before.

'It could come at any time,' said Julia.

It was Friday evening – twenty-four hours since David had said that she might have no more than two hours.

The bedroom door had developed a harsh squeak every time anyone came in or out. Rosemary whispered to Elizabeth: 'That door. Have you any oil?'

Elizabeth nodded and left the room. Again the door shrieked a hideous protest.

A few minutes later there was another squeak and Elizabeth returned with the familiar injection tray.

'Thank you, Elizabeth.' Julia held out her hand for the syringe.

'No, no!' The note of horror in Elizabeth's voice stopped Julia short, her hand outstretched. 'That's not for Jane. It's the oil for the door!'

Rosemary hoped that Jane was still able to hear what was going on. It was the odd spot – the moment of ridicule in the middle of tragedy – that her daughter would have appreciated.

Julia and Elizabeth were smiling. 'I hope you don't use the syringe on the patients after this?' Rosemary said.

'They're usually thrown away. This is an old one,' Elizabeth reassured her in case she really was worried.

Frank, the porter, asked if he could come in to say good-bye. He stood holding Jane's hand for several minutes, then turned to us. 'Thank you,' he said, and left the room in silence.

June in England is a time of long evenings. The light doesn't fade from the sky until around eleven o'clock. It was midsummer night. The neo-druids would be gathering for their vigil on Stonehenge, waiting for the dawn rays of the sun to rise between the old stones and strike the place they believe was the ancient altar.

Their old friend, Sue, had come to be with Rosemary. She stayed late into the night talking while the sound of Jane's harsh breathing filled the room. They spoke of Jane's childhood and of the war years. It was strange to remember a time before she had been born. During the past five months the struggle to cope with her illness and the fear of defeat had been uppermost in her mother's mind. Remembering the years before Jane's life had begun helped Rosemary to deal with the idea of her death.

About two o'clock on Saturday morning, Rosemary pressed the bell, and Emily, on night duty, was in the room in an instant.

'Her breathing has changed,' said Rosemary. 'Suddenly . . . now it's so quiet I can't hear anything unless I get very close.' She watched as Emily leaned over Jane. 'Does this mean it's nearly over?'

Jane lay like a marble statue of death on a medieval tomb, white and still. Her arms were crossed over her chest. Her hands bent at right angles to her wrists. Her breathing was almost inaudible.

Emily straightened her back and smiled quietly. 'She still has some way to go.'

As the day began, Jane's quiet breathing persisted. The pulse at her throat was calmer. It was a surprise to the doctors and nurses that she struggled on so long, but it wasn't a struggle, merely a continuing, a going on. There was no hint of pain or stress. Her face was serene; her limbs seemed completely relaxed.

During the day the outer rim of her lips began to show white. Then, slowly, this area of pallor increased until her mouth was as pale as the rest of her face. Only her hair, brows and lashes showed colour.

Julia suggested that from now on we should stay in the building. She arranged to have our lunch brought to the room.

The last rose of Jane's life was picked from the garden outside her window. There was only one flower growing in a bed of neglected bushes. It was a white bloom, just beginning to loosen from the tight bud, without the slightest flaw on either petals or leaves. Rosemary cut the stem with surgical scissors. A single drop of dew lay in the fold of the petals. The bud was pure white, without a fault, a perfect rose. Too perfect, Jane would have said, almost too good to be true. Rosemary laid it on Jane's pillow, close to her face.

The signs of death were clear. Her flesh was shrinking into itself more rapidly. Hour by hour her body became softer, thinner, limper, more fragile; deep lines and white patches showed where it had rested against the bedding. Talking softly to her as they turned her over, the nurses rubbed her skin where the patches showed, soothing the bruised flesh.

The last time they turned her it was as if there was no life in her body, no resistance to the pressure of the arms that lifted her.

Victor was on the terrace when Jane's breathing suddenly changed to a high thin note, infinitely sad and far away. Rosemary felt she had heard this sound before somewhere. It carried an unmistakable warning. But she hesitated to call Victor.

Then the sound of Jane's breathing changed again. This time it was low and soft, each breath so light it could scarcely be heard. Rosemary called Victor.

We stood on either side of the bed, each holding one of her

hands. As we listened, the breaths came lighter and lighter. Jane's head moved very slowly, as if reaching up for air, and her eyes were open a fraction, showing a slit of light.

Then everything was still. There was nothing more. The pulse at her throat had ceased.

We have seen pictures of the dead who died violently – victims of murder, accident, war. These are the terrible images etched into our minds: the distorted bodies of those who died in pain and fear.

For us, who watched Jane's quiet end, there is a memory of her still, peaceful face and the warmth of her skin beneath our lips as we kissed her goodbye. This slow, gentle death was a natural end to life. The waning of her body was easy to believe and to accept. Her retreat had been strangely beautiful to watch. We felt no fear.

Epilogue

We had a promise to keep.

'It'll be a fun place for my ashes,' she had said of the garden of Dairy Cottage. It was a hard thing to do, to open the small box and to touch the pale, grey powder. We kept putting it off. But one morning as the sun broke through the clouds and the garden came to life after a heavy rain, with the grass glistening and the water lily opening its petals in the warm light, we both knew that the moment was right.

We walked through the grounds arm in arm, remembering the places she liked best: the grassy slope she used to lie on to catch the sun, the pond where she would sit for hours watching the fish and the moorhen, the stream where she used to play with Richard. We thought of how Jane had walked there for the last time, just after Dr. Sullivan had told her the truth. As we retraced Jane's steps, we halted at the places where she had stopped as if she had been trying to fix them in her memory. We took handfuls of ash and scattered them in an arc through the air, like a peasant scattering the seed. We threw them on the flower beds, under the old yew trees, over the water. The wind blew the particles in a wide circle as they fell. Little flakes settled on the roses. The soft powder lingered on the surface of the pond, near the willow tree Jane had helped to plant, before sinking slowly to the bottom. Then it was all gone.

We cried a little. But Jane had begged us not to mourn her. 'I don't want anyone to be unhappy because of me.' That was all very well, one of her friends had said, wiping a tear, but it wouldn't be easy.

It took a few weeks to organise the party that Jane wanted.

She said it was to be a happy party, to make up for the birth-day she had missed while she was ill. She had given some thought to the invitation list: her friends, she said, and all the people who had helped us during her illness. Everyone came – Dr. Sullivan, the Brighton bank manager who had given his time to a project that never materialised; the families who had opened their homes and their hearts to us when Jane needed human warmth between hospitals, not a rented flat; the hospice people who were not on duty that Saturday afternoon; and, of course, Jane's young friends. One of them had said, 'It will be a vegetarian meal, of course.' This seemed to create a huge problem because many of the guests were meat eaters and might not enjoy the food that Jane's own crowd liked. Would it spoil the party for them? Could Rosemary cook the dishes that had been Jane's speciality? But the problems melted away when several of Jane's friends announced they would come to stay for the weekend. They would cook, help to get the house and garden ready, prepare the punch.

So it happened that the party began long before it was due to start, as the best parties do. The kitchen was full of cooks. In the hall the punch was mixed without a recipe but with plenty of ingredients and a lot of enthusiasm, and another group was arranging tables, chairs, benches in the garden. In the middle of it all a neighbour arrived, barely visible behind a huge bucket full of roses from his garden – tall-stemmed flowers, strong and healthy, with many blooms to each stem. 'Would you like some more?' he asked, and soon the whole house was full of colour and scent. Roses lay on the tables, on the chairs, on the floor. Everybody had heard about the rose Jane wore in her hair until she died. The hospice people talked to her friends about the Jane they knew at the end, and learned from them about the younger Jane they hadn't known. Victor spoke briefly, insisting that Jane was in no way special, that surely her friends knew that—it was the hospice alone that had made her peaceful end possible. She had been there only eight days, but they had been days full of life, full of meaning.

It was a good party. There were no tears. People broke up into small groups and talked not only of Jane but of dying, of how it can be made bearable, of their own fears and hopes. Her friends were happy for Jane and proud of her. There were none of the stilted formalities and embarrassed condolences of a funeral. This was not a wake. It was a cheerful thanksgiving, not just because Jane had wanted it to be so, but because she had provided the theme that made this possible.

When we went back to Washington at the end of the summer, we became aware of a change in ourselves. We were thinking far more than ever before about what really matters in life, about feelings, about the more abiding human values, about people – people as individuals. Jane talked of all these matters in her last weeks, and she made them more real to us than they had been. She also took pleasure in passing on her more cherished possessions to her friends. She gave a lot of thought to it. She liked to see them walk away with something she had given them, after they had said goodbye.

'I don't need a "thing" to remember Jane by,' said one of her friends. 'Jane taught me how to make bread. Whenever I make bread, I think of her.'

Before she died, we had talked of how people live on in what they do, in their actions, in the memories of those they have influenced. That was how Jane hoped she would live on. And she will.

A great deal still remains to be done to extend the scope of care for the dying and to enhance its standards. Jane's parents believe that an important role in accomplishing this could be played by the establishment of university Readerships and Chairs in Hospice Studies. They are making an initial contribution from the royalties on this book for the endowment of such a Chair, and any readers who wish to associate themselves with this effort may do so by sending their own contributions, earmarked 'For the University Chair', to the National Society for Cancer Relief, 30 Dorset Square, London NW1 6QL.

VOLUNTARY HELP. *Hospices are grateful for many kinds of voluntary help. If you live near one (see page 250) and think you can help, please get in touch. You can also join an initiative group (see page 252), or work to start one in your area.*

Afterword

There are thirty or forty hospices in Britain at the time of writing, in 1980, but more are being planned. By no means all those dying of cancer or other diseases need a hospice, for in many cases the terminal stages are less painful or distressing than is generally imagined. But there still remains a large number of people who need help and don't know how to go about getting it.

The best way to apply for admission is through the patient's general practitioner. He is likely to know what hospices exist in the area, and will usually make the necessary arrangements. However, some doctors are not yet persuaded of the benefits of hospice care, and may be reluctant to help. When this happens, the patient or the family should insist on a second opinion, or a third, and in the last resort can approach their area health authority. Most hospices are run by the National Health Service; private hospices usually have arrangements with local health authorities so that anyone can be admitted regardless of their means.

The initiative in starting a hospice is usually taken by a local group. The National Society for Cancer Relief in London, which has played a major role in establishing most hospices and home care services, stands ready to help such groups with organisational advice and funding when appropriate. In the past the objective was usually to build a separate unit, and this would then be handed over to the National Health Service which would take care of its running costs. This, however, tends to be looked at askance by some consultants, who fear that it may divert money from the hospital beds needed by their patients. And the increasing success of hospice home care teams is showing that more can be done for less money, and is reducing the demand for hospital beds. The first step now is usually the setting up of a home care service which may in time lead to the establishment of a residential hospice.

Most patients want to die at home, and a hospice team will do everything they can to make that possible. The home care unit can provide the patient with many of the services available at the hospice. Above all, the patient and the family know they will not be abandoned just because no further curative treatment is available. The members of the team, doctors and nurses, social workers and clergymen, therapists and voluntary workers, will help to handle any medical, emotional, or financial problems, however serious or petty they may seem. The nurse can teach the family how to take a more active role in looking after the patient. At a time of stress she will usually become aware of the undercurrents that flow through the family, of its strengths and weaknesses, and will be able to help marshal its resources for the struggle. She will often act as a mediator, a link between members of the family who may find it hard to communicate, a repository of confidences and complaints, and finally as a friend who is always there to help, a lightning rod for the inevitable outbursts of anger and frustration.

At home the team can help members of the household more easily than at the hospice to cope with the stress of bereavement, the feelings of loss and guilt, which may be alleviated by the active role the family is taking in caring for the patient. The grief of parting may be eased for both patient and family if they have been able to work through it openly in the intimacy of the home. When death takes away the member of the family who dealt with the day to day problems of living, financial, legal, and the like, the hospice team will provide advice, not just sympathy, or will find out where the necessary help can be obtained. 'It can be difficult to find someone to talk to,' a nurse will tell the bereaved. 'Come back to us whenever you want to. We'll always be here.'

But although much of the hospice work can be done more effectively at home, this does not mean that the need for the residential unit will disappear. There are always the more difficult cases that cannot be taken care of at home, the terminally ill without a family, and those who need a bed for a few days now and again to give the family a rest. Far too many patients now arrive at the hospice in extremes of pain which could have been avoided through earlier admission. A timely assessment by a home care nurse could prevent this kind of deterioration by treatment at home, but it could also determine that the patient's condition requires the thorough and extensive study that is best carried out in a hospice. After this the patient could go home, and return to the hospice only if a further change made it necessary for his condition to be re-studied, and his treatment adjusted. This is increasingly the pattern of hospice admissions.

Residential hospice units are also necessary as centres for teaching and research. Nor is it only prospective hospice workers who could benefit from such training. Few physicians practising today have been taught how to care for the dying. Because all the emphasis in their training and work is on how to cure people, they often regard a patient's death as a failure, a personal defeat. The teaching of hospice skills and attitudes must become an important and fully integrated part of the university curriculum. The lack of such training is a disgrace, and it is the dying who pay for it. It is high time to establish university chairs in hospice studies and the care of the dying which would provide the focus for both teaching and research.

The hospice movement is not an organisation with leaders, branches, and paid up members. It is a community of people who have been touched by death, who know that it can be made more tolerable, and who are determined to make it so. It has arisen spontaneously, first among the nurses and physicians who followed in the footsteps of Dr Cicely Saunders (now Dame Cicely), who established the first modern hospice in London in 1967. She trained the first generation of hospice workers and has travelled to many countries spreading the word and setting an example, so that there are now between 400 and 500 hospices in the world.

The hospice movement is gaining a growing number of adherents as more and more of us come to see that the increasing complexity of modern life, a culture that sweeps death under the rug, and a technology that becomes an end in itself, deny us the human and humane end which our nature demands. Nothing can ever remove the grief of dying, but hospice care can make death less fearful, more acceptable. Hospice offers the gift of living, paradoxical as this may seem, to both the patient and the family, and ultimately to society as a whole. For it enables us to share in the dying of those we love in a way which helps us to change our own attitude and thus to change the attitude of others.

The humanisation of medicine implicit in the hospice approach need not and should not be confined to the treatment of the dying. The de-personalisation of medical care as a whole is a process that must be halted and then reversed. Here, too, the hospice is showing the way. It has something of importance to teach all of us, for few people are likely to go through life without having to face a life-threatening crisis of one kind or another. We are all afraid of dying, to a greater or lesser degree. We all want our fears to be eased, and to relieve the fears and pain of those we love, and in this sense we are all members of the hospice movement.

LIST OF HOSPICES

This partial list of hospices is based on information compiled by Barry Lunt of Southampton University. The National Society for Cancer Relief, Michael Sobell House, 30 Dorset Square, London NW1 6QL (telephone: 01-402-8125), will be pleased to give further information.

* denotes hospices with home care units. † denotes hospices or home care services founded or supported partly or wholly by the NSCR and bearing the name Macmillan.

Avon †* The Dorothy House Foundation, 162 Bloomsfield Rd, Bath BA2 2AT.

†* St Peter's Hospice, Tennis Rd, Knowle, Bristol.

Cheshire †* St Ann's Hospice, St Ann's Rd North, Heald Green, Cheadle, Cheshire.

Cornwall †* Macmillan Home Care Service, Truro (home care only).

Dorset †* Macmillan Unit, Christchurch Hospital, Christchurch.

Hampshire †* Countess Mountbatten House, Moorgreen Hospital, West End, Southampton.

Kent   * St Bartholomew's Hospital, Symptom Control Team, Rochester.

†* Care Foundation, Michael Tetley Hall, Sandhurst Rd, Tunbridge Wells.

London   * The Hostel of God, 29 North Side, Clapham Common, SW4 0RN.

The Horder Ward, Royal Marsden Hospital, Fulham.

†* St Joseph's Hospice, Mare St, Hackney E8 45A.

* St Christopher's Hospice, 51 Lawrie Park Rd, Sydenham SE26 6DZ.

St Thomas' Hospital, Symptom Control Team, Lambeth Palace Rd, SE1 (home care team only).

Manchester   †* St Ann's Hospice, Peel Lane, Little Hulton, Worsley, Manchester M28 6EL.

Middlesex   †* Michael Sobell House, Mount Vernon, Northwood.

Midlands, West   †* St Mary's Hospice, Raddlebarn Rd, Selly Park, Birmingham 29.

Norfolk   †* Priscilla Bacon Lodge, Colman Hospital, Norwich.

Northants   † Cynthia Spencer House, Manfield Hospital, Northampton NN3 LAD.

Nottinghamshire   †* Hayward House, City Hospital, Hucknall Rd, Nottingham NG5 1PB.

Oxfordshire   †* Sir Michael Sobell House, Churchill Hospital, Headington, Oxford.

Staffordshire   † Douglas Macmillan Home, Barlaston Rd, Blurton, Stoke-on-Trent.

Surrey   †* Sam Beare Ward, Weybridge Hospital, Weybridge.

Phyllis Tuckwell Memorial Hospice, Trimmers, Waverley Lane, Farnham.

† Kingston Hospital, Macmillan Symptom Control Team, Kingston (home care service only).

Sussex   †* King Edward VII Hospital, Douglas Macmillan Continuing Care Unit, Midhurst.

Sussex, East   Copper Cliff Nursing Home, 74 Redhill Drive, Brighton.

Sussex, West   St Barnabas Home, Columbia Drive, Worthing BN13 2QP.

Yorkshire   †* Wheatfield Hospice, Wood Lane, Headingley, Leeds.

  * St Gemma's Hospice, Leeds.

  †* St Luke's Nursing Home, Little Common Lane, Off Abbey Lane, Sheffield.

  Wakefield Home Care Service, Wakefield.

Scotland   †* Roxburghe   House,   Tor-na-Dee   Hospital, Aberdeen.

  †* Roxburghe House, Royal Victoria Hospital, Dundee.

  †* St Columba's Hospice, Challenger Lodge, Boswell Rd, Edinburgh.

Wales   † Macmillan 'Mini' Units (2 hospice beds plus relatives' bed-sitter per unit).

  Amman Valley Hospital, Ammanford.
  *Brynseiont Hospital, Caernarfon.
  *Groeswen Hospital, Port Talbot.
  Monmouth General Hospital, Gwent.
  Oakdale Hospital, Blackwood, Gwent.
  S. Pembrokeshire Hospital, Pembroke Dock.
  Treherbert Hospital, Rhondda.
  Royal Denbigh Infirmary, Denbigh.

LIST OF INITIATIVE GROUPS

Cheshire   St Rocco's Hospice Project, Mr F. Howliston, Hon Secretary, 4 Hillford Crescent, Walton, Warrington, Cheshire.

Cleveland   Middlesbrough Continuing Care Service, Colin Dickinson, Area Administrator, Cleveland Area Health Authority, Marton House, P O Box 92, Borough Rd, Middlesbrough, Cleveland TS4 2EI.

Devon   St Luke's Hospice, Plymouth, Campaign office, c/o Computer Services (South West) Ltd, Millbay Rd, Plymouth PL1 3NG.

Essex   St Francis Hospice, Mrs Joan A. Gornall, The Hall, Broxhill Rd, Havering-Atte-Bower.

Herefordshire   The Freda Pearce Foundation, Dr R. G. Miller, 8 Norton Ave, Hereford HR2 6DN.

Humberside   North Humberside Hospice Project Ltd (Home Care only), Hon Secretary, 11 Ashgate Rd, Willerby HU10 6HH.

Kent   East Kent Hospice Project, Mrs S. Rawlings, Summer Hayes, Cliff Rd, Hythe, Kent.

Wisdom Hospice, Rev D. S. R. Redman, The Rectory, 65 Maidstone Rd, Chatham, Kent.

Lancashire   Continuing Care Unit, Lancaster, Mrs L. Parker, Acting Secretary of the Steering Committee of the Board of Trustees, Thwaite Gate, Carnforth, Lancs LA5 9EL

The Wigan Hospice Project, The Rev E. Rowlands, Chairman, Haigh Vicarage, Coppers Lane, Wigan WN2 1PA.

Lincoln   The St Barnabas Hospice Project, Organising Secretary, The Rookery, Chapel Lane, Heighington, Lincs.

London   Hospital of St John and St Elizabeth, Matron, 60 Grove End Road, London NW8 9NH.

Merseyside   Wirral Hospice Project, Dr J. A. Aitkin, Consultant Physician, Clatterbridge Hospital, Clatterbridge Rd, Bebington, Wirral, Merseyside L63 4JY.

Mid Glamorgan   Bridgend Hospice Project, Mr P. V. Davies, Area Administrator, 18 Cathedral Rd, Cardiff CF1 9SJ.

Sussex   Macmillan Domiciliary Service, Hastings Health District, Dr J. S. Plumpton, Consultant Anaesthetist, Royal East Sussex Hospital, Hastings, Kent.

Macmillan Domiciliary Service, Eastbourne Health District, Dr Joan B. Hester, Consultant Anaesthetist, District General Hospital, Kings Drive, Eastbourne, E Sussex BN21 2UD

Stirlingshire   Strathcarron Hospice Appeal, The Rev Tom Scott, Appeal Director, Randolph Hill, Fankerton, by Denny, Stirlingshire.

Tyneside   St Oswald's Hospice Ltd, A. C. Taylor Esq, Hon Secretary, 86 Pilgrim St, Newcastle upon Tyne.

Wiltshire   Prospect Foundation Ltd for Continuing Care, Rev M. D. Evans, Chairman, 7 Temple St, Swindon.

Yorkshire   St Leonard's Hospice, Chairman of St Leonard's Hospice Appeal Committee, Grimston Hill House, York YO1 5LE.

Calderdale Society for Continuing Care, Mr J. Taylor Secretary, Flat 8, Sallerville, Skircoat Green Rd, Halifax.

MARY

by Patricia Collins

A CHILD YOU'LL WANT
TO REMEMBER.

Mary Collins was a really beautiful baby. Born
prematurely, she had a tiny oval face, a rosebud mouth
and an enchanting smile. The third child of parents who
came from the bustle of New York to make a home in
Ireland, Mary found a warm and secure place in the heart
of the family.

**Then, eight months later, Patricia Collins learned
that Mary was brain damaged. Doctors diagnosed
cerebral palsy; she would probably never walk
and she would almost certainly be retarded.**

The shock of this discovery plunged Patricia into despair.
Mary needed extensive therapy and the burden of caring
for her increased Patricia's growing resentment and guilt
– she began to drink heavily, blaming herself for what
had happened. When circumstances forced the Collins
family to return to America, Patricia made a wrenching
decision to leave Mary behind in Ireland in a residential
home for two years. The years in Ireland did nothing to
lessen the severity of Mary's disabilities, but another kind
of change did occur. Mary was becoming a determined,
courageous child with a winning personality and she
gave a very special purpose and meaning to life.

This is an intimate, inspiring and deeply moving account
of a mother's journey from despair to joy and of the
power of the human spirit to overcome adversity through
love and understanding.

A STORY YOU WON'T FORGET.

BIOGRAPHY   0 7221 2482 1   **£1.50**

A SELECTION OF BESTSELLERS FROM **SPHERE**